PRAISE FOR COLLEGE LIFE OF A RETIRED SENIOR

"Blackwood's story of returning to college as a senior citizen is so vivid and inspiring, you might find yourself compelled to start looking at course listings, no matter your age. An amazing tale of determination and resilience, told with humor and grace."

—Marcia Trahan, author of the memoir *Mercy*

Yvonne Blackwood chronicles her years balancing her pursuit of a university degree with an active life as a senior. Although this memoir will be of special interest to English Majors, woven through the story are strategies useful to anyone contemplating post-secondary education. Through perseverance and dedication, Blackwood overcame obstacles posed by a global pandemic and her own health challenges to graduate *Magna Cum Laude*.

—Laurie Ness Gordon, Author of *The Medal and Finding Home*

Blackwood's million-dollar question on how she will manage her established lifestyle and attend university and the soul searching that followed, set the stage for any reader of this book to continue to see how well she fared and whether she persevered to the very end.

—Gloria Wilson-Forbes, Retired teacher

ALSO BY YVONNE BLACKWOOD

Into Africa:A Personal Journey
Will That be Cash or Cuffs?
Into Africa the Return
Nosey Charlie Comes to Town
Nosey Charlie Goes to Court
Nosey Charlie Chokes on a Wiener

COLLEGE LIFE OF A RETIRED SENIOR

A MEMOIR OF PERSEVERANCE, FAITH, AND FINDING THE WAY

YVONNE BLACKWOOD

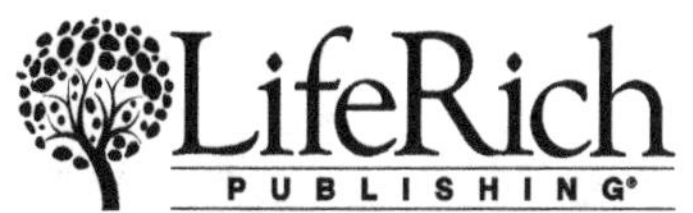

LifeRich Publishing books may be ordered through booksellers or by contacting:

LifeRich Publishing
1663 Liberty Drive
Bloomington, IN 47403
www.liferichpublishing.com
844-686-9607

ISBN: 978-1-4897-4637-5 (sc)
ISBN: 978-1-4897-4635-1 (hc)
ISBN: 978-1-4897-4636-8 (e)

Library of Congress Control Number: 2023902291

Print information available on the last page.

LifeRich Publishing rev. date: 03/06/2023

Dedication

To my son Robert, your love and assistance is much appreciated
To my grandsons Theo and Anthony, set
your sights on higher education.

Contents

Preface

The world of universities and the world of retired seniors seldom overlapped. I was determined to merge both for a few years, at any rate. The world of retired seniors can be as vibrant as an exercise club or as dull as a graveyard. But humans were given free will. We all have choices. You determine which world you want to inhabit.

I retired from a thirty-seven-year banking career months before my fifty-seventh birthday. I had lived my life setting goals and working to achieve them and had implemented one in the 1980s to retire at fifty-five. When I finally handed in my retirement notice a couple of years later than the original goal, but with good reason, I planned to spend more time writing.

I published my first book, *Into Africa: A Personal Journey*, in 2000 and my second book, *Will That be Cash or Cuffs?* in 2005 while working full-time. During the writing, publishing, and markcting of these books, I wrote articles for three newspapers and published short stories in anthologies. I was in the throes of writing my third book when I retired.

Although I planned to devote more time to writing after retirement, I insisted that it would not prevent me from doing more of the things I loved. I planned to travel more, entertain friends and family more, go to the theatre more, and read more. But people come into our lives for a reason and a season. Influencers have a way of appearing like genies without warning or explanation. It is up to us to recognize them and determine if we want to travel the path they try to lead us.

I was a member of The Writers' Union of Canada (TWUC) for several years. In 2013, the organization suggested that members could form small writers' groups if several lived in a local area. I did not know it then, but several writers lived in Richmond Hill, where I resided. They met and formed a group with the blessing of the TWUC representative in the province.

I attended the inaugural meeting, where I met Olga, a seventy-five-year-old author and former journalist. Olga and I exchanged copies of our books. Two months later, at the second meeting, Olga said she loved my story and recommended I pursue an English degree at York University. "I have that degree, and it has helped me to add texture to my writing. It will do the same for your writing," she said. At first, I was annoyed with her for giving unsolicited advice; however, I overcame the annoyance when I realized that she could be right. I had always felt that my writing was not textured enough. Perhaps earning the degree would help.

I pondered Olga's suggestion over several months, and the more I thought about it, the more the potential benefits of attending university appealed to me. In addition to improving the texture of my writing, other strong reasons came into focus. Dementia was ravishing more and more senior citizens daily. In his book *Chasing Life*, Dr. Sanjay Gupta wrote, "The prospect of memory loss is so unnerving because we are, in many ways, the sum of our memories…memories tie us to our past, to our family and friends and to the events that shape our lives." Research showed that exercising the mind could ward off the terrible disease called dementia. I figured that pursuing studies at the university could help avert it.

Plus, humans are social beings. Attending university would give me a reason to get dressed and leave the house a couple of days each week to be with other people. It would provide a consistent structure for several years.

The fourth reason was to inspire my two young grandsons: to show them that you can learn at any age, and to encourage them to aim to attend university after high school.

I would have loved to devote most of my time to pursuing the degree, but I didn't want to neglect the other duties I had committed to—sitting on a government board and three committees, being the head teller at my church, and occasionally babysitting my grandsons. I wished to avoid stress but keep my life balanced, so I gave myself six years to earn the degree. My flaw was my discipline, my conscientiousness, my persistence, and my habit of intense hard work. Those foundations of resilience helped me maintain the quality of life essential for survival.

One of the great things about going back to school when you are a senior is that you relearn things you have learned before, only this time, myths are dispelled. You suddenly realize, goodness gracious, that was incorrect all along! For example, there was no Trojan horse in *The Iliad.*

I hope *College Life of a Retired Senior* provides an incentive for others, especially retired folks like me, to return to school and pursue courses, even a degree, or pursue goals you once dreamed of but have put aside. Do not be deterred by retirement. I could have dressed up this story and made it look easy, but I wanted to be honest. Many millennials earned their degree easier and faster than I did. Of course, there were times when I wished my brain were sharper, my memory quicker, and my joints stronger—no arthritis. But as my darling grandmother used to say, "If you want good, your nose must run."

During my studies, I forged through the fog, trying to find a way, and stumbled upon hurdles, including two strikes—one lasting five months; the COVID-19 pandemic; hard-to-connect-with millennials; and the highest one—a diagnosis of sarcoma cancer in my right thigh. I stayed the course because of my faith in God and strong support from family members, my church family, and my fabulous friends. Pearl Bailey said, "Go for it, Honey," when she encouraged seniors to pursue studies. I am thrilled that I went for it, that I took on the challenge, that I tried the way (*Tentanda via*), that I climbed the mountain, and that I graduated magna cum laude from York University. I say this: nothing is easy, perseverance and determination are excellent qualities, and success is sweeter than the honeycomb. Pursue your ambition with gusto. Go for it!

CHAPTER ONE

Why Go Back to School Now?

"Develop a passion for learning. If you do, you will never cease to grow."

—ANTHONY J. D'ANGELO

"Why go back to school now?"

"What do you plan to do with the degree when you receive it?"

"Are you planning to teach?"

I was taken aback by several of my friends, both men and women, when they asked these questions after I informed them that I was pursuing an English degree at York University. I had merely expected to hear, "Oh, that's wonderful," or "I wish you all the best with your studies. Let's celebrate when you complete it." Human reactions always amazed me.

Perhaps the person who surprised me most was my father. Dad was eighty-nine at the time, with a mind as sharp as a scalpel. He lives in Florida and regularly had positive, animated conversations with me on the phone. He would quote scripture I'd read and long forgotten. Unlike many seniors his age, who tended to talk about the good old days, Dad always talked about current affairs. He would rattle off details about the happenings in the United States and the current political issues. He loved baseball and kept up-to-date with the major teams. When I told him I was pursuing an English degree at university, he said, "Why bother to do that now? You already did your studies." The tone of his voice emitted disapproval. I suppose he thought having two of my siblings, his children from a second marriage, currently attending university was enough. They were the ages of my two oldest grandchildren, so perhaps he thought it was odd for me to be in university while they were. I decided to say nothing more about my studies unless he asked. I let his lacklustre response fizzle and changed the subject.

At age sixty-four, I had accomplished much. Career-wise, I had worked in the banking industry for thirty-seven years. I held positions with The Royal Bank of Canada that included bank manager, community banking advisor, and commercial credit advisor. As a writer, I am an author, columnist, and award-winning short story writer. As a community volunteer, I have been president of Tropicana Community Services Organization—Toronto's largest black community service organization. I have been a board member and secretary of the Metro Toronto Children's Aid Society, a board member of the Ontario Development Corporation, a board member of the Trillium Foundation, and a mentor with the YMCA Black Achievers Program (to name a few positions). I'm presently a board member of the College of Nurses of Ontario. As a traveller, I'd established a goal to set foot on six of the seven continents (being a hot-blooded woman, Antarctica didn't interest me). I had achieved that goal by travelling all over the world.

Having done all that, I could sit back on my derriere and do nothing, but I do not view life that way. My philosophy is: as long as you have health and strength, there are always new dreams to fulfill, new horizons to explore, and new mountains to climb. Einstein said it aptly, "Once you stop learning, you start dying." According to York University's Faculty of Liberal Arts & Professional Studies, the study of English literature develops critical thinking and communication skills necessary to excel in life and your chosen career. I looked forward to acquiring those skills—not to excel in life or a career, but because I craved knowledge. Obtaining an English degree was the latest mountain I planned to climb, and like Sir Edmund Hillary, I was determined to reach its summit.

There is a story behind my decision to eventually register in the English degree program at York University at this time. My college days were back in the early 1970s before I immigrated to Canada from Jamaica. I remember those days fondly. Young and vibrant, I emitted energy and had an excellent memory. I only had to read a text once, then review it before the exam. Today, I have to read a text at least twice and review it twice. My memory is no longer what it used to be. Yet I've never forgotten Miss Johnston, my economic geography teacher. Forty-five, attractive, and unmarried, she was outspoken and loved to counsel her students. I recalled the day she returned our first exam papers, and one girl burst into tears because she had received a mark of 65 percent for her effort. With a glint in her eyes, Miss Johnston said, "My dear girl, nothing is wrong with reaching for the stars, but if you can't reach the stars, take the ceiling, nuh!" I liked Miss Johnston, but I did not accept that advice. I preferred, "If at first you don't succeed, try, try, and try again."

I intended to abide by the creed I had lived by from childhood, the creed that is forever in my mind, the creed that has helped me to succeed in life despite many obstacles. The words of Henry Wadsworth Longfellow: "Perseverance is a great element of success. If you only knock long enough and loud enough at the gate, you are sure to wake up somebody." I was determined not to allow an aging lazy memory or anything else to deter me from obtaining an English degree.

In the 1980s, racism jumped up and nicked my face like a discontented cat in Canada, and promotions in the banking world moved slower than molasses in February. I concluded that my

Associate of the Institute of Bankers diploma from Cambridge University was not good enough, that I had better pursue the Canadian banking diploma, so off to night school I went. Within three years, I obtained the Fellowship of the Institute of Canadian Bankers (FICB) designation. I believe it helped me along the path to promotions. I had not attended any institute of higher learning since the early 1990s except to take two short, specialized courses.

While working full-time at the Royal Bank, I published my first book, *Into Africa: A Personal Journey,* in 2000. Becoming an author had been a wonderful experience, and my employer supported me well. I was a community banking advisor at that time. The branch manager of the building where I had my office organized a book signing party for me. I can still visualize the big square cake with the image of the book cover etched into it. My boss and two vice presidents attended and made sure to purchase autographed copies of the book. I subsequently published *Will That be Cash or Cuffs?* in 2005 and *Into Africa: The Return* in 2009.

After that, I joined The Writers' Union and have remained a member. I had little interaction with the members. The Annual General Meetings were hosted in different cities across Canada each year. I attended the meetings held in my city, Toronto, and on those occasions, I interacted with some members. I don't know what spurred the union to make a change after operating the same way for years, but in 2013, they recommended that members could form small writers' groups if several of them lived in the same vicinity.

Writers in Richmond Hill, where I lived, quickly formed a group. I attended the inaugural meeting, held at a popular restaurant in the area. At the small group meeting, I met and became instantly friendly with Olga, a seventy-five-year-old woman with platinum blond hair, blue eyes, and well-defined lips. We were the first to arrive, and while waiting for the others, we chatted. She was sharp as a new razor. She seemed keen to read my travel memoir, and I was interested in reading her book on autism, so we exchanged copies of our books.

The group held a second meeting two months later. When it

ended, Olga pulled me aside. "Yvonne," she said, her voice dripping with syrup, "I finished your book, and I enjoyed the story very much. I like your writing style. You know what I would do if I were you?"

"What?" I asked abruptly. My antenna flew up like radar. I detest people who offer unsolicited advice, especially when I don't know them very well.

"I think you should do the English major degree at York University. Your English is excellent, but I have that degree, and I find it helps me to add texture to my writing. I know it will do the same for your writing."

My eyes stopped flashing.

I calmed down.

Okay, I could accept texture.

I've always felt that my writing needed more depth, more layers; yet, despite all the writing courses that I had taken and the myriad of books I had read about writing, I had not mastered the art of texture. I thanked Olga for her suggestion and promised to think about it. I later learned that she has five degrees, including two PhDs. I deduced that if anyone knew about texture, she did.

Learning to add texture to my writing became the primary reason for pursuing an English degree at York U., but I had other strong reasons also. I'd read that acquiring knowledge through lifelong learning—like a new dance, speaking a foreign language, or writing newsletters—can truly benefit senior citizens. These benefits include keeping your mind sharp, improving your memory, and increasing self-confidence. I had no issue with self-confidence; I exuded it. But as mentioned before, my memory was not as sharp as it used to be.

Memory loss was exploding in the seniors' community, and although none of my friends had dementia, we were concerned it may develop in us. I had read *Chasing Life* by Dr. Sanjay Gupta. In it, he wrote, "When you're sixty-five, there's a one in ten chance you are affected by Alzheimer's. By the time you're over eighty-five, there's almost a one in two chance you have the disease." It was a quote from the Alzheimer's Association. Gupta also quoted Scott Hagwood who said, memory is something we need to work on; it's like a muscle.

* * *

My posse of six ladies, all of Caribbean heritage, and all divorcees except one, had been meeting annually for dinner on the Saturday closest to Valentine's Day over several years. Each one took turns hosting the dinner. It was always a lavish spread. The host would cover the dinner table with a red tablecloth and set it with her best crockery (a throwback from our Caribbean upbringing), sparkling crystal glasses, exquisite flatware, and red cloth napkins. All the ladies wore something red—a dress, a skirt, a blouse, a jacket, or a scarf. Those occasions were lively, filled with laughter, and continued beyond midnight.

In recent years, the subject of memory loss inevitably surfaced at our gatherings. At the most recent dinner, Ada, the funniest lady in the group, ushered in the topic by saying, "Lord, ladies, my CRAFT [Can't Remember a Fucking Thing] is getting worse every day." She then added an anecdote about one of her recent memory-loss incidents. The rest of us chimed in and shared our memory-loss stories. Although we laughed at the stories, they forced me to think. What if these small memory losses represented the beginning, and we were spiralling toward dementia? I felt that pursuing a degree, especially one loaded with literature, would be a perfect antidote, a way to exercise my brain muscles as suggested by Scott Hagwood.

The third reason for pursuing the degree was to provide me with ongoing, consistent structure for several years. Attending university would compel me to get out of bed, get dressed, and leave the house at least twice each week, rain or shine. It wasn't that I remained in bed most of the day; I did not. During the first two weeks of retirement (I retired early), I slept in, feeling no need to arise early, with no job to go to, and nothing specific to do by a certain time. I discovered something alarming. My days became so short I had practically no time to do anything. How could I live the rest of my life this way?

I immediately reverted to setting my alarm clock again. I would set it for 7:30 instead of 6:30, the time I'd set it for when I worked, and rolled out of bed by 8:00 a.m. After that, my days became long, I accomplished much, and my retirement life became fulfilling. My home was a delightful sanctuary, but sitting around all day, even if I spent most of my time writing, was not stimulating enough. And yes, I spent time reading many cases to prepare for meetings at the College of Nurses each month, but my third-term appointment would end in less than two years. I would have extra time on my hands, time that must be channelled toward something meaningful.

The fourth reason was to inspire my two young grandsons: to show them that you can learn at any age. Watching the news over the years, I noticed that many black youths had gotten into trouble with the law. Most of them had not pursued education beyond high school. I did not want my grandsons to fall into the trap of "the system." My son and daughter had done courses at college, but they had not gone full-time to a university. They had obtained average jobs. In recent years, a paradigm shift occurred. A grade twelve education used to be the basic requirement for a job. Today, an undergraduate degree had become the standard for a good-paying job. I wanted my grandsons to follow in my footsteps and attend university full-time. As the adage states, "Children live what they learn."

CHAPTER TWO

Exploring Campus

"The idea of being with my peers at a real school seemed much more exciting than making movies"
—SHIRLEY TEMPLE

After York U. accepted me into the English degree program, it suddenly dawned on me that I knew little about the lives of university students in the twenty-first century. I would be attending classes, some in the mornings and some in the afternoons, with the regular day students. What did the students wear? How did they carry their books? What amenities existed on campus?

I didn't want to wait for the beginning of the school year in September; instead, I planned to begin my studies in early January, the start of the winter semester. I had visited York U.'s main campus on Keele Street a few times when I'd taken two courses there more than twenty years ago. I attended those courses at night after my workday ended and had no time to explore the campus. I went from my car to the classroom, to home. On another occasion in 2001, I visited the campus as a guest on CHRY, York U.'s radio station.

Luther Brown, one of the radio hosts, had interviewed me on air about my travel memoir, *Into Africa: A Personal Journey.* Those days were long gone. I suspected that the campus had changed significantly. I set aside a day to explore it before the winter semester began.

I arrived on campus on a Wednesday at 9:00 a.m. Established in 1959, York University is Canada's third-largest university. Its main campus at Keele and Jane Streets occupies more than one square kilometre of land. Precipitation was mild that morning, and a thin layer of snow had already covered the ground. I drove around searching for parking and was surprised to discover that the campus had several parking lots; however, only a few were assigned to students. Most lots dedicated to student parking were far away, and you had to walk a long distance to the buildings. The price of parking made me suck in my breath. Signs on the little green parking metres stated $1.50 per half hour or a flat fee of twelve dollars per day. A quick calculation told me that attending any course that lasted three hours would cost almost the flat fee. How could poor, struggling students afford to park here? I decided then and there not to drive to campus. I would explore public transportation; it must be much cheaper.

Later, I searched online and discovered that my senior citizen status allowed me a fare discount of almost 50 percent. I started to like my senior status more and more as perks materialized. I learned that a York Region Transit (YRT) bus travelled along Yonge Street from Newmarket, veered west onto King Road, near where I lived, and then travelled south on Keele Street, west onto Steeles Avenue, and directly onto the campus. I printed the bus schedule. It showed that buses arrived at my stop—a mere seven-minute walk from my home—every twenty minutes. My senior's discounted fare was $2.10 one-way, less than it would cost to park for one hour at the university. I had not travelled by public transportation for many years; it would become my weekly mode of commuting to York U.

On that exploratory Wednesday morning, I parked my car as close to one of the buildings as I could, then walked gingerly along the snow-covered ground to a paved path leading to Central Square.

I headed to Vari Hall, where a permanent information desk stands. The students manning the desk were helpful and answered all my questions. I collected a small map of the campus grounds, showing the buildings, streets, and parking lots. I placed the map in my wallet. It served me well over the years as my classes took place in classrooms located all over the campus.

After leaving the information booth at Vari Hall, I lingered along a corridor where hordes of my fellow students stood around talking and laughing. They were brown, black, and white. Years earlier, when I was heavily involved in community work, I learned that Toronto is one of the most multicultural cities in the world, and that people from more than 160 countries reside there. York U.'s students reflected multicultural Toronto. I stopped now and again to observe the students and listened in on bits of conversation. I made a mental note of the garbs female students wore—jeans, T-shirts, sweaters, and hoodies. I had slung my handbag over my shoulder but noticed that no one else carried one. Everyone had backpacks on their backs. I watched as some students took off their packs and put them back on with ease. *Oh brother, when will I be able to do that without making a fool of myself?* I had never owned a backpack. Some girls—the more fashion-conscious ones—wore boots with high heels, but most wore running shoes. Although winter raged, no one wore long coats. Bomber jackets and short puffy coats were the standard. I made another mental note to inspect my closet, then go shopping before attending my first class.

I entered The Scott Library, the main library on campus, and took a cursory look around. Its large structure spanned five floors and housed thousands of books. From the main floor with "The Ask Us Desk," escalators ran up and down, taking you to all the levels. If you didn't want to use the escalators, a bank of elevators on the right would take you to any floor. I took the escalator to the second floor and stepped off onto a wide, open area. There were no books here, just chairs, tables, computers, and an information desk. The man at the desk explained that I could use one of several computers in the area to learn which floor to find a book, but of course, he could help me to do that. I knew then that in the coming years, I would spend much time in the library, if not physically, then online.

It was important to know where to find food since some days, I would have two sessions of classes and would not wish to worry about sustenance. I learned that you could purchase food in small cafeterias located in some of the major buildings or from vending machines placed in most buildings. But York Lanes is the hub. It has a large two-story food court where you can sit, relax, and enjoy a hot meal. Popular fast-food restaurants like Wendy's, Popeyes, and Pizza Pizza are on site. Dozens of cultural groups living in Toronto operate small restaurants here too. You can purchase Thai, Indian, Greek, Middle Eastern, and Caribbean cuisine any day of the week. I sampled the Caribbean food that day—jerk chicken, rice and peas, and a scoop of creamy coleslaw. I was satisfied with it and would return to The Islands Caribbean Restaurant numerous times during the six years I attended classes on campus. Frankly, I should have owned shares in the company by the time I completed the degree.

My campus exploration ended with a visit to the York U. bookstore. Located at one end of York Lanes, the bookstore occupied two floors. I entered the first floor and found it brimming with books at one end, a vast array of school supplies in the middle, and clothes, drinkware, and souvenirs in another section. Clothing included T-shirts, sweats, jackets, and hoodies. Souvenirs included mugs, water bottles, and glasses, all embossed with York U.'s logo and name. I bought several medium-sized notebooks since I planned to take copious notes during lectures. I also bought all the supplies I thought I would need for my first semester.

I took the stairs to the lower level, and discovered a labyrinth of shelves stocked with all the textbooks and reading materials suggested by professors. I couldn't quite figure out the shelf labelling. To avoid wasting time (the parking metre was ticking), I asked a student clerk to help me find the textbooks for my English course. He led me to a section with shelves stocked with textbooks for all English courses. Labels with course names and numbers hung above each shelf. Textbooks, new and secondhand, were stacked below, allowing you to choose which one to purchase. I'd never bought a secondhand book but thought it might be a good option, especially for the more expensive textbooks. I flipped through a few and observed some passages highlighted with yellow or orange markers, underlined sentences and paragraphs, and pen-written notes at the side of some pages. No, this would not work for me. I intended to do my own underlining and highlighting. I opted to purchase, all new, the textbooks required for my first course. I would return to the bookstore semester after semester to purchase my books. I also returned when the store held sales, which were often, to buy some of the embossed clothing and souvenirs.

On the way home, I deviated from the main path and drove to a mall, where I purchased my first backpack. I had no experience putting one on or taking it off, but I'd observed the students on campus. Resolute not to embarrass myself, I practiced putting it on and taking it off, standing before the full-length closet mirror. I was determined that when I stepped onto the YRT bus, I would whip off my backpack with ease, and when I stepped off the bus, putting it back on would be a breeze.

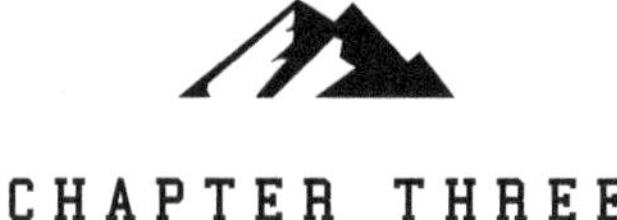

CHAPTER THREE

I Wouldn't Abandon My Former Life

"Great achievement is usually born of great sacrifice, and is never the result of selfishness."

—NAPOLEON HILL

Before I embarked on my journey to earn the English degree at York U., I had already spent seven years as a retiree. During those years, I enjoyed a satisfying, rewarding life. I'd ramped up my travels to twice each year, ticking off the places I visited from my bucket list. I'd been on the board of the College of Nurses for several years, with less than two years to complete my final appointment. Sitting on the council of the College, plus three other committees, gobbled up a good chunk of my time each month. The work proved interesting, and I learned firsthand about Ontario's health care system, which I suspected I would eventually utilize, but hoped the time wouldn't arrive for many years. Little did I know, it would be sooner than I expected.

Being a woman of faith, I served the Lord and by extension, my church. I was the head teller. Besides collecting the offering plates from the ushers on Sundays, placing the offerings in canvas bags, and locking them in the vault, I spent every Monday morning at the church office with another member (joint custody), counting, recording, and balancing the offerings collected at both services on Sundays. After we balanced the books, we drove a short distance to the bank and deposited the funds. My church hosted a gathering on Thursdays lasting two hours, dubbed LAFF—Life After Fifty-Five—for seniors. A moderator welcomed everyone, guided the first hour by telling a few jokes (clean ones), led with a couple of hymns, and introduced the guest speaker, who would talk for about twenty minutes. After that, the audience headed downstairs to enjoy a hot lunch. The pastor and I alternated as moderators every other week. I intended to continue those church activities.

I was the emergency babysitter for my two young grandsons and called upon occasionally to do just that. I intended to remain available, just not on my school days.

While I worked full-time, I hosted large, fun get-togethers, but they had a downside: I never spent much time with individual guests. After retiring, I changed my entertainment strategy to hosting small, intimate luncheons with four or five people. Attending university wouldn't deter me from hosting these luncheons; however, I would host fewer.

I had been keen to maintain close contact with family members and good friends after retiring. Today, some of my dearest relationships are with friends from my high school. I planned to keep those relationships intact.

The million-dollar question was, how would I manage my student life and maintain my established lifestyle? I decided that I would not carry a full course load each semester. My goal was to obtain a degree for my edification and not to earn it quickly to find a job. I planned to take it nice and slow. I gave myself six years to obtain the degree, expecting to reward myself with a grand seventieth birthday present in 2020. I even had the celebratory event meticulously planned in my mind: I would rent a banquet hall to accommodate sixty friends and family members. The affair would be a formal sit-down dinner. Linen tablecloths and napkins would grace the tables, and champagne would flow freely. My son, Rob, would produce a short video encapsulating the main highlights of my life from childhood to graduating from York University. It would include clips from my work life, community volunteer life, family life, church life, travel life, and friendship life. The event would end with a couple brief, poignant guest speeches and my thank-you speech. Oh, it was going to be a grand celebration.

I decided not to take any courses scheduled on Mondays to avoid clashing with my church work. In the end, I had to do a few classes on Mondays—clashes were unavoidable. My teller partner graciously accommodated me by switching those Mondays to other days. I appreciated him for that.

I needed to take at least one summer course every year, preferably a six-credit or a nine-credit class, in order to complete the BA in six years. I intended to continue to travel, but would have to do so during free time between semesters. There were roughly three free weeks between the winter semester ending in April and the summer courses beginning in May, and three weeks available between the summer courses ending in early August and the fall semester commencing in September. When the fall semester ended in December, about three weeks remained free before the winter courses began in January. The available times restricted when I could travel to avoid missing class time. But in life, you must be flexible and work around situations to achieve your goals. In other words, you can have your cake and eat it too, but perhaps not the entire cake.

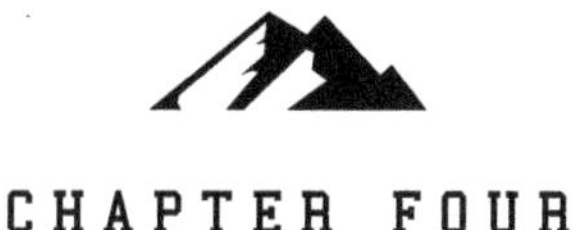

CHAPTER FOUR

Commuting to Campus

The first class of my first semester at York University was scheduled to start at 11:30 a.m. I was commuting from home and wanted to arrive on campus an hour early. I had lived in the suburbs, in the town of Richmond Hill, in the region of York, north of Toronto, for twenty years. The block of my street, just north of Lake Wilcox, interposed by a section of the Oakridge's Moraine, a natural habitat for birds and other animals, was a little paradise. Living here felt like living in the country, but the city still breathed down your back.

Giddily, as if I were going on a shopping spree, energetic in the early morning, I headed out to York U. from my quiet townhouse complex at 9:30 a.m. I bundled up in a thick, short black winter coat with the hood covering my head, the legs of my jeans tucked into new short leather boots, a woollen scarf wrapped around my neck, and my hands clothed in thick woollen gloves. My new backpack rested comfortably on my back, loaded with textbooks, a notebook, pens, pencils, a water bottle, and a small makeup bag. I placed my Presto card in my coat pocket for easy access. I walked along the private road of the townhouse complex to the main street, then proceeded west to where it met Yonge Street at a set of stoplights. A fire station stood at the left. I crossed Yonge Street to the west side and passed a drugstore and a garage selling tires. The sharp, cold January air caused my nose to run. With my arthritic knees, it took me seven minutes to walk to the bus stop. The bus arrived on time, and I entered the classroom an hour before the class began. I would repeat that walk every season for the next six years.

* * *

York Region has its own transit system (YRT), separate from The Toronto Transit Commission (TTC). The busses connected with the Toronto Transit Commission service at some terminals. If you wanted to go downtown via public transportation, you had to pay two fares. That was not the case for me to attend York U. I took only one bus. York Region had implemented the smart card automated fare collection system called Presto in the summer of 2011. Since I had never travelled by public transit at that time, I was unfamiliar with it. In preparing to attend York U., I quickly read up on the system and applied for the card. Having a Presto card in my wallet meant I didn't have to worry about carrying the correct fare in cash. I merely stepped into the bus and tapped the card against the Presto box near the driver. A ding sounded, the machine deducted my fare, and that was all. The system knew my card belonged to a senior and collected the discounted fare. My job was to make sure my Presto account had sufficient funds. The Presto system made it easy for commuters, allowing them to add money to their card online any time from the comfort of their homes—a great convenience.

At first, I thought of my commute as merely getting to York U., as traversing the space between Richmond Hill and the university, but over time, I came to think of commuting as absorption into the environment. Soon I began to lap up the view and observe commuters. The bus stopped at every stop along the way. After a forty-five-minute drive (if weather and road conditions were good), it entered the university campus and deposited student passengers a short walk from York Lanes. It then turned around and headed for the terminus.

During my time at York U., I made sure to catch the YRT bus that would deposit me on campus at least an hour before my classes started. I was never late for a class. Having worked in the corporate world for thirty-seven years, I had been chiselled and moulded into a punctual zombie, and a stickler for punctuality. After I had attended York U. for several weeks, the drivers recognized me. One male driver always smiled at me and said, "Good morning, miss." I naturally smiled back at him and said, "Good morning."

The buses were never full, so I always had a choice of seats. On the way to class, I used the time to reread the text for the day or review an assignment I'd completed, always making sure to be prepared for my classes. On the way home, I used the time differently. I relaxed and tried to unwind, watching the traffic zipping by, listening in on conversations of commuters (a habit of writers), sometimes jotting down actual conversations. If I attended an evening class, I would sit by a window and watch the sun sink in the west, its dying rays streaking the sky in orange and fuchsia. I did not mind commuting at all.

As the bus headed toward campus, I loved to look around and try to guess who the passengers were. During each semester, when classes took place on the same days, I encountered some of the same people. I knew their stops and in which buildings they worked. Commuters minded their own business and rarely made eye contact with me.

Ten or more York U. students usually rode the bus, depending on the time of day. They would rush off like a herd of buffalo as the bus pulled up on campus. It seemed they never allowed themselves extra time as I did. Even when I tried to keep in step with them on the short walk to York Lanes, I was always the last to enter the building.

I'll be forever grateful to York Region Transit for its reasonably reliable public transportation. It saved me hundreds of dollars in gasoline bills during the six years I commuted and watched gas prices fluctuate from ninety-seven cents per litre to almost two dollars per litre; it saved me countless dollars in parking fees had I driven to the campus and the dread of driving on snow and ice-covered roads in winter. But the most enjoyable part of commuting was sitting back in my seat mornings and evenings, reflecting on my studies and watching the world go by.

Writers are always interested in sceneries. I'm no exception. As the bus travelled along King Road, I observed that the small bungalows, built probably before the 1950s, were slowly being replaced by modern two-story houses. Builders who'd acquired three or four bungalows, demolished them and constructed a row of two- or three-story townhouses in their places. These townhouses, built close to the road, had no front yards. At Keele Street, near Highway Seven, commercial and industrial buildings with colourful signs advertising their products dominated the landscape. Many people worked in those buildings, and the YRT was the means of transportation for many of them.

I observed the seasons change and display spectacular vistas. The bus traversed along main roads, then snaked its way through quiet residential areas with well-appointed middle-class homes where children played in small community playgrounds. It passed parklands with lush verdant vegetation in the summer and yellow and orange foliage in autumn.

In the summer, parts of King Road and Keele Street sported gorgeous baskets of colourful flowers hanging on lampposts; some sat on the sidewalks. It was delightful to travel this route at Christmastime, when decorative lights replaced the hanging baskets of flowers, and many residences and commercial buildings exhibited multicoloured lights with various themes.

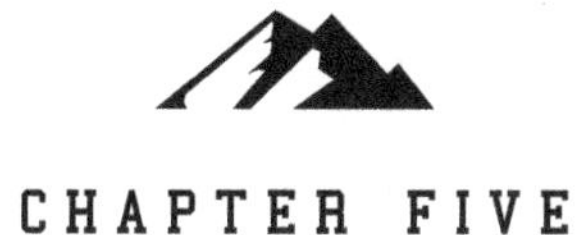

CHAPTER FIVE

A Smorgasbord of Things to Learn

"I've always loved the first day of school better than the last day of school. First are best because they are beginnings."

—JENNY HAN

The Academic Calendar for the Faculty of Liberal Arts & Professional Studies spelt out clearly, in black and white, the requirements to earn an English degree. Besides obtaining the mandatory thirty credits in English courses, you must obtain six credits in natural science, and nine credits of approved general education courses in the social science or humanities categories, and six credits approved in general education courses in the opposite category to the nine-credit course in social science or humanities already taken. You also had to obtain a GPA of at least 4.00.

The word "science" in natural science made me nervous. "I know little about science," I moaned. The last time I took a science course was during my high school years, many moons ago. The subject was biology. I had been keen to learn about human anatomy, but the day I had to dissect a frog, I ran out of the lab with my hands covering my mouth. How could I earn a passing grade for natural science courses? The little voice inside my head (it is always there in times of stress) said, "Calm down, Yvonne, have faith." Moments like that, when doubt swirled around me, I recited my go-to Bible verses: "Trust in the Lord with all thine heart, and lean not unto thine own understanding. In all thy ways acknowledge him, and he shall direct thy paths." These verses have given me much strength over the years. I calmed down and focused on the two compulsory English courses that were prerequisites to proceeding with the degree.

The humanities include the study of languages, literature, history, the arts, and philosophy. It made sense to pursue studies in this field to obtain an English degree. I looked forward to exploring all or some of those areas.

Social science is the branch of science devoted to studies of societies and the relationships among individuals within those societies. The field included subjects like economics and politics. I had been a banker all my working life, so economics naturally interested me. I became actively involved in politics in the 1980s when Alvin Curling, a black brother, decided to run as a provincial member of Parliament. A groundswell of grassroots campaigners sprang up to help. I was one of them. I remained interested in politics at the macro level. I felt that exploring courses in social science should prove stimulating.

It mattered not which courses I had to take; I was hell-bent on obtaining the English degree, convinced by my colleague, Olga, that it would help me to add texture to my writing. York U.'s motto is *Tentanda via*, "the way must be tried." Whatever proved to be the way, I intended to try it. What I didn't know was how much the pursuit of the degree would inform me, challenge me, satisfy me, and drive me to consider giving up on more than one occasion.

* * *

I arrived at Curtis Lecture Hall #H one cold January morning, bundled up in my new, short black winter coat, a chunky sweater, a woollen scarf wrapped around my neck, my hands clothed in thick woollen gloves, and my new backpack on my back. I was an hour early as planned. No other students had arrived. I chose a seat in the third row and placed my coat and backpack on the chair beside me. I whipped out my notebook and a pen, placing them on the desk. While waiting, I reread Rebecca Solnit's essay, "The Faraway Nearby."

Professor Blazina entered the room ten minutes before class time. He was a short man with a scraggly beard and a moustache, bald from the mid-back of his head. He wore a green army-type jacket, a black V-neck shirt, and grey corduroy pants. He seemed like someone ready to retire. He spent the first few minutes fiddling with the equipment at the front of the room in preparation for the lesson. More than sixty students had filled the hall when he began to lecture.

I was attending Introduction to Literary Study. The course outline specified that it would train students to observe, understand, and evaluate how literary texts are written and how to write effectively about literature. Three teaching assistants (TAs) supported the professor. They attended to make sure the tutorial discussions that would follow the next day connected with the lecture. During the semester, I attended classes with Professor Blazina on Thursdays and tutorials with Michelle, my TA, on Fridays. She was a petite girl, about twenty-four, with silky black hair and big, bright eyes.

Five minutes into the lecture, Professor Blazina became extremely irritated by students who insisted on keeping their cell phones on. He may have been ready to retire, but his hearing was by no means impaired. He heard every ping on the cell phones when text messages arrived. He stopped speaking, slowly surveyed the room, then said, "Listen to me. I think your parents are paying good money for you to be here. They didn't put a gun to your head. I didn't put a gun to your head, so if you don't want to be here, you can go."

He waited.

Silence filled the room. No one got up to leave.

He continued the lecture.

At one point, Professor Blazina placed a slide with a list on the overhead. I was quickly jotting down the items when a male student sitting at my left held up his cell phone and snapped a picture of the list as if it were the most natural thing to do. I looked at him, and if looks could kill, he would have been stone-cold dead. I was a notetaker. The thought of snapping a picture of the professor's notes never crossed my mind. I was sitting there, writing until my fingers were about to fall off, and this boy merely snapped a picture. "You little bugger," I thought. "So, this is how the young ones do it." I was sweating, trying to copy the list before the professor changed the slide, and all he did was snap. Would he even look at the picture again? Would he read it for his review? I consoled myself that my way was better, that once at home, I would reread the list and type it. Repetition helps to retain information, and I needed to improve my retention skill.

Since most students used their laptops, tablets, or cell phones during the lectures, they continued to annoy Professor Blazina. In the midst of a lecture another day, he asked, "What is it with this texting? Is it an addiction?" Rhetorical questions, I suppose. A sprinkling of nervous laughter enveloped the room. The addicts knew who they were.

If you are sociable, you quickly discover that making friends with peers is almost impossible during lectures. Students packed into lecture halls, and everyone faced forward, the goal being to pay attention and listen to the professor. If you sat in the middle of a row, you could converse with students on either side, but you had better not during the lectures. When classes ended, students rushed out like the room was on fire, either to their next class, to tutorials, or to the library.

How do you get to know your classmates or make friends if not during lectures? You do so in tutorials held in more intimate settings with fewer students. Most tutorials I attended had desks arranged in a square. It allowed students to make eye contact with each other and talk directly to their classmates even if they sat across the room.

Tutorials were designed to facilitate discussions, and here you heard students speak and share their opinions. You soon discover who is opinionated, a wise guy, withdrawn, or a sourpuss. Michelle, my teaching assistant, began the first tutorial by going around the room and asking each student to say something—their names, current university year, their major, and something interesting about themselves that no one could guess. This exercise became the modus operandi for teaching assistants throughout my studies.

Some students provided so much detail you wanted to say, "Shut up, enough already." I always kept my introduction short and gave little information about myself. I deliberately NEVER mentioned that I'm a published author or a retired banker. I merely wanted to be a regular student pursuing an English degree and did not want to attract any attention to myself.

* * *

York U. views academic cheating very seriously. Before submitting my first paper, I logged into the university's website and read a tutorial on academic integrity. After that, I completed the Academic Integrity Quiz, consisting of ten questions. Every student must answer all questions correctly or repeat the quiz until they score 100 percent. I read the tutorial carefully, making sure I understood the lessons. I scored 100 percent on the first try. I printed the document showing my score and kept it in my files for future reference.

Professors made it their duty to remind students about plagiarism. A paragraph in the syllabuses addressed academic honesty in every course I took, reminding us that plagiarism can lead to charges of breach of academic honesty.

Some universities, including York U., now insist that students submit their papers via Turnitin. According to its description, Turnitin is a plagiarism detection system that compares files students submit against its database and produces a similarity report and score for each assignment. I thought it galling that students would copy other people's work without ascribing them credit and try to pass it off as their work. But this is the real world in which we live. Students did it all the time, and some get caught and kicked out of universities.

The day came in Professor Blazina's course when students had to write their first essay. The assignment asked us to compare and contrast two of the short stories we had read. He instructed us on what he expected. Adhering to the instructions, I selected two stories, reread them, and analyzed them, then wrote my essay. I edited and reedited the essay, and polished it as best I could, then submitted it to Michelle, my TA. Two weeks later, she returned it graded. I received a C+. Now, a C+ was a good mark for some students, but it devastated me. How could I, a published author and a conscientious student who adhered to the lessons taught, receive a C+? Besides, I'd set a goal that my marks should never be less than a B.

I took a deep breath. No, I took several deep breaths, and assessed the situation. Alright, I had published three adult nonfiction books, three children's picture books, several short stories, and numerous newspaper articles. But had I ever published any essays? No. The essay is prose that you can enhance with literary devices like similes, metaphors, and anaphora. It is its own genre with its own rules and structure. The compositions I'd written in college in the 1970s were a far cry from today's essays. At the university level, you must adhere to the rules. I concluded that perhaps I should learn more about the genre before pouncing on Michelle, a graduate student with a lot of experience writing essays.

I ate a chunk of hard-to-swallow humble pie and made an appointment to meet with Michelle. I arrived at her office, a little cubbyhole in the Ross Building. Michelle appeared apprehensive when I walked in, waving the essay in my hand.

"Poor girl," I thought. "Let me put her mind at ease."

"Hello, Michelle," I said, "I'm not here to beat up on you about my marks. I'm sure you have a good reason for giving me a C+. I'm here for you to tell me what I need to do to improve my marks going forward."

Michelle exhaled, and I heard the air leaving her lungs and travelling all the way into the atmosphere.

"Oh, thank you, Yvonne," she said. "I'm having a hard time with some of the students. One boy even threatened me if I don't change his marks."

I was shocked to hear this. Imagine a student, probably Michelle's age, threatening her about marks instead of trying to find ways to improve them. Back in my college days, students wouldn't even look directly into the eyes of teachers, much less threaten them. To do anything of the kind would show the world that you were ill-bred, ill-mannered, and impolite. No one wished to wear such a bull's-eye on their back.

I consoled Michelle and told her, "Do not allow students to bully you. Just make sure the marks you give are fair and justifiable. And by the way, report the student who threatened you. No one should be threatened for doing an honest job."

After that, Michelle and I sat side by side at her little round table and dissected my essay.

"Your thesis statement is very good, but some of the subsequent paragraphs defending it have some weaknesses," she explained.

We scrutinized each paragraph, and she pointed out where I could improve them. I concurred with most of her points. As we reviewed the last paragraph, the conclusion, Michelle reiterated what Professor Blazina had said:

"You take your introduction and essentially say to the reader, 'See, I told you so.' It should say strongly that you have proven everything you had set out to prove."

I thanked her and left the office with an air of confidence, thinking adamantly, "You, missy, will never, ever give me another C+."

Introduction to Literary Study was all-encompassing. Professor Blazina examined the genres of short stories, poetry, drama, and essay. He never missed a class and always arrived on time. He blew his top a couple more times during the semester about the same thing—students preoccupied with their electronic devices and not paying attention.

The last time he became angry about the texting distraction, he said, "I should go out in a blaze of glory!"

A blaze of glory! What would that look like? My vivid mind sprang into action. I visualized Professor Blazina dressed in a black leather suit and a black cowboy hat, sitting atop a white horse. He prodded the horse with the silver spurs of his black boots, and the horse charged from the lecture hall. The image captured the attention of students who kept peering at their cell phones, and they dashed out of the room after the professor. The white horse charged down the corridors of Central Square, through to the hallways of the Ross Building, through Vari Hall, and exited the hall through the front door into the courtyard. A mob of students following stopped short as the horse jumped over the oval fountain and galloped into the sunset. I returned to reality and heard Professor Blazina say, "We will discuss sonnets next class."

During the poetry segment, Professor Blazina lectured on sonnets. We examined the Petrarchan, Spenserian, and Shakespearean sonnets. He challenged each student to write a sonnet in any of the three types, promising that he had five books to award as prizes for the best attempts. From a class of over sixty students, only three of us took on the challenge. I crafted a Shakespearean sonnet, convinced it was the easiest of the three types. I couldn't believe that my first-time attempt was all that good when I won first prize. Slim pickings, I suppose. For my prize, Professor Blazina gave me a book on literary terms. The book helped me as a reference in other English courses I subsequently studied.

Near the end of the course, Professor Blazina disclosed that he planned to retire, confirming my earlier thoughts. When the course ended, the class had dwindled by one-third.

* * *

I tried to recapture the spirit of my old college days and settled into my studies in my first year at York U. I attended workshops conducted by the Learning Skills Services. They widely advertised their calendar of workshops for each month on the campus. I figured that in this twenty-first-century digital world there must be something new and helpful I could learn to make my studies easy. The first workshop I attended was Reading and Note Taking. Since I habitually took notes longhand and typed them afterwards, I was keen to learn a new method that was less laborious. Lessons from the workshop confirmed what I already knew: the more you handle your notes, the more you will remember them. I did not learn much more.

I still felt I could benefit from the workshops and attended another, Time Management. I'd worked in the corporate world for thirty-seven years and held management positions where time management was crucial to meeting deadlines and addressing many time-sensitive matters. I was disappointed in the workshop and regarded it as tame. It taught me nothing new; however, I would recommend it to students just coming out of high school; they would benefit from it. They say that experience teaches wisdom. My work experience taught me how to manage time. I applied that knowledge to my study time. I never attended another Learning Skills workshop.

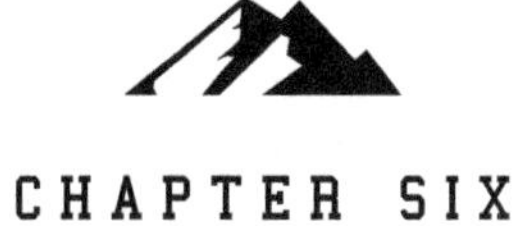

CHAPTER SIX

Exploring Africa American Literature

"Without language, one cannot talk to people and understand them; one cannot share their hopes and aspirations, grasp their history, appreciate their poetry, or savor their songs."

—NELSON MANDELA

It was all well and good that I had taken English courses that explored British Literature. But as a black student, I would have been negligent if I had not studied some types of black literature. I mentioned earlier that I was born and raised in Jamaica, an island the British captured from the Spanish in 1655. The British imported slaves from Africa and shipped them to the Caribbean Islands, including Jamaica. By the end of the seventeenth century, most of the population of Jamaica was black. The British modelled Jamaica's education system after their system. In primary and high schools, students studied the works of famous British authors and poets like Charles Dickens, Robert Louis Stevenson, and William Wordsworth.

I always smiled, noting the irony, when I recalled primary school students reciting,

> I wandered lonely as a Cloud
> That floats on high o'er Vales and Hills,
> When all at once I saw a crowd,
> A host of golden Daffodils…

None of us had ever seen a daffodil at the time. Although most of the population is black, we never studied black history or literature by blacks.

Jamaica lies relatively close to the United States (only a ninety-minute flight to Miami from Montego Bay) yet, African American literature was never taught in schools—at least not while I lived there. Of course, I later learned about the concept of divide and rule. Plato said, "Better be unborn than untaught, for ignorance is the root of misfortune." But the airwaves roamed freely, and we picked up American stations on our radios. Later, when television arrived in the island, American shows became our dominant programs. I loved soul music. Aretha Franklin and many black male groups like The Temptations, The Four Tops, and The O'Jays overshadowed the airwaves in the late 1960s and 1970s. Jamaicans became absorbed in African American music, but no one made a concerted effort to teach students African American literature.

After immigrating to Canada in the 1970s, I had easy access to books written by African Americans. Works by Maya Angelou, Walter Mosley, Terry McMillan, Alice Walker, and Toni Morrison sit prominently on my bookshelf today. While listening to discussions about slavery on American television stations, I realized that the African American experience was much different from that of the blacks in the Caribbean. Knowing this, I decided early in my studies at York U. to explore African American literature. I wanted to gain a more scholarly insight about their authors, poets, and artists to dispel any myth I may have harboured over the years.

I registered for African American Literature. The short

description of the course stated, "The course provides an introduction to African American literary movements and traditions from its origin to contemporary twenty-first-century literature."

At the beginning of the fall semester in 2014, I arrived at a Vari Hall classroom for my first class. The professor was an attractive, stylishly dressed African American woman. She explained to the students that she would teach the course in a three-hour format, integrating lectures, class discussions, and oral presentations by every student. She would evaluate us based on quizzes, supervised tests, essays, research projects, unsupervised take-home exams, and our oral presentation in class. Professor Alston provided a document with a more detailed course description. It specified that we would explore the origins of African American literature, which included vernacular, work songs, the blues, folktales, and slave narratives, to name a few.

I sensed that I was in for a treat.

"Bring it on. I'm ready to climb this mountain," I thought. "I'm ready to learn."

The primary textbook for the course was *The Norton Anthology of African American Literature.* Chock-full of essays, manifestos, poetry, plays, speeches, and excerpts from novels, it contained 1,574 pages, including selected bibliographies and indexes. I was pleased to see that one of the general editors was Henry Louis Gates, Jr. He was on PBS's *Finding Your Roots.* In our first three lectures, Professor Alston delved into the early history of African American literature. As I took more English courses, it became clear how literature and history are intertwined. African American Literature is about writings by black Americans. The questions I asked were: Why does it have a category of its own? Why is it unique?

Professor Alston provided the answers as she took us on a journey that traversed the byways and highways of African American literature. We explored the when, where, why, and how this literature came about, grew, and transformed over four hundred years.

When: The first enslaved Africans arrived in America in 1619.

Where: Slaves were bought and sold mainly in the Southern states.

Why: Slaveholders were capitalists who bought and sold slaves like horses. Slaves were chattels, and the owners were white supremacists. Slaves in the South were not allowed to read or write. They used vernacular tradition, which is oral, and which was their only way to communicate. Some slaves in the South learned to read until a law prohibited them. Slaves in the North, in places like New England and New York, were allowed to read and write. Acquiring literacy proved to be a powerful weapon. It revealed that the theory some whites held, that Negroes were inferior, would be thrown out if they were allowed the opportunity. Through the writings of blacks, common humanity became authenticated.

How: In the early years, slaves sang songs—work songs—as they carried out their tasks. Later, educated slaves began to write their autobiographies, called slave narratives. Phillis Wheatley was the first slave to publish a book in the 1760s; however, the first slave narrative, *The Interesting Narrative of the Life of Olaudah Equiano, Or Gustavus Vassa,* was published in 1789 in London. He was captured at age eight with his sister by his countrymen in West Africa and moved from place to place until they sold both to white men who shipped them to the New World. Equiano provided good insight into his life as a small boy growing up in West Africa. He expounded on family unity, different tribes, and languages that were easy to learn. He described the stench and horrible conditions onboard the ship that took him from Africa, his adult life in England and other places, and how he survived while enslaved until he purchased his freedom in 1766. Equiano wrote his story at the start of the abolition movement and used it as a primary text to plead with the white establishment to abolish slavery.

The slave narratives are powerful. As I read Harriet Jacob's *Incidents in the Life of a Slave Girl* (published 1861), tears tumbled down my cheeks. How could white men who claimed to be civilized behave in such uncivilized ways? Jacob narrated her struggles so dramatically, you could not help feeling sympathy for her and wishing that she would become totally free of her slave master.

Paul Laurence Dunbar became one of the first influential black poets in American literature. He was acclaimed internationally for his dialectic verses, published in *Majors and Minors* (1895) and *Lyrics of Lowly Life* (1896). Dunbar had to write in vernacular because the patrons of his works were mainly white, and they wanted that sort of speech. The irony was that he was not a Southerner and did not know the Southern talk well. But the patrons wanted Southern pastoral, so he provided it.

Professor Alston continued with our journey through decades of African American literature and arrived at the period labelled The Harlem Renaissance. It lasted from 1919 to the 1940s.

Encyclopedia Britannica describes The Harlem Renaissance this way:

> A blossoming of African American culture, particularly in the creative arts, and the most influential movement in African American literary history. Embracing literary, musical, theatrical, and visual arts, participants sought to reconceptualize "the Negro" apart from white stereotypes that had influenced black people's relationship to their heritage and each other. They also sought to break free of Victorian moral values and bourgeois shame about aspects of their lives that might, as seen by whites, reinforce racist beliefs.

Alain Locke, a black intellectual during that era, introduced some poets to white patrons. Patronage helped them focus on their craft without worrying about paying bills; however, it had a downside. Langston Hughes eventually cast off his patron when she insisted that he write blacks as "primitive." The black intellectuals tried to direct writers how they should write. At that time, W. E. B. Du Bois was editor-in-chief for the NAACP. He criticized any book that did not portray African Americans positively. But writing, art, and theatre are developed from individual creativity, and no person can or should control what a writer can write. The educated African American writers wrote successfully in several genres. During The Harlem Renaissance, Contee Cullen crafted his famous poem, "From the Dark Tower," as a Petrarchan sonnet.

At the end of the lectures on The Harlem Renaissance, Professor Alston gave us an assignment that we had to present to our classmates. Each presentation was to last a maximum of half an hour, with a few minutes extra for questions and answers at the end. Each student chose the day and time to present. I selected the fourth slot.

I was the old senior in the class who had given many speeches over the years. As president of a community service organization, I delivered speeches to its members and the public in general. As a community banking advisor, I addressed businesses. As an author, while promoting my adult books, I had addressed several audiences using *Into Africa: A Personal Journey* as a catalyst to encourage people to pursue their dreams. My audiences included Rotary clubs, high school and college alumni associations, community organizations, and even two large hospitals in New Jersey. The words *stage fright* had evaded my vocabulary. Presenting to my classmates with the professor observing would be a breeze.

I chose the subject for my presentation and researched it. I typed my document with a sixteen-point font, double-spaced, which allowed me to easily read it while glancing up and making eye contact intermittently with my classmates. I rehearsed the speech at home, and timed it to make sure I stayed within the limit.

The classroom was furnished with long tables arranged in a square, with chairs placed around them. A small table and a chair for the professor stood at the front centre of the room, and a podium stood in the front right corner.

The first three presenters arrived at class with their written documents. They sat in their seats at the long tables and read their presentations without drama, with their heads down, without making eye contact with their classmates. The presentations were informative, but the deliveries were dull and pathetic.

On my presentation day, I did not sit in my seat. I stepped up to the podium at the front of the room, the spot where Professor Alston usually stood to deliver her lectures. I figured that a little parody would attract and hold the attention of my peers and began my presentation this way: "Friends, Canadians, countrymen, American!" (I turned toward Professor Alston when I said, "American.") "Lend me your ears! I've come today to talk about The Harlem Renaissance, and in particular, to spotlight two writers involved in the movement."

Laughter filled the room.

My classmates became instantly engaged.

They were ready to listen.

I stated that the presentation would be in three parts: an overview of the period; an essay titled "The Harlem Renaissance—Langston Hughes and Countee Cullen: Vernacular or Classic Format, a Matter of Opinion," and the reading of a poem. I looked directly at my peers from time to time and outlined the phenomenon of The Harlem Renaissance, mentioning that it encapsulated visual art, music, fashion, theatre, prose, and poetry. I then read the essay. In it, I described James Weldon Johnson's disappointment that African Americans had discarded traditional dialect in their poetry. He felt that they would regret it. I compared Langston Hughes and Countee Cullen, two very successful poets who proved Johnson wrong. Their works proved that black poets could become successful whether they wrote in vernacular and embraced black subjects like Hughes did, or wrote in a classical genre like Cullen. I ended my presentation by reading "Mother to Son" by Langston Hughes. I pointed out that Hughes used vernacular style and wrote in free verse but applied several literary devices. I opined that the poem is really an extended metaphor, with life equated to a staircase. I bowed at the end of my presentation. The room erupted with applause. I distributed handouts with listings of the works of Hughes and Cullen.

A male student rushed to the podium. He said, "I love your presentation. Do you mind if I borrow your style?"

"Oh, please go ahead. If it makes your presentation better, use it. Always remember, eye contact is important," I said.

The students departed, and as I gathered up my paperwork and leftover handouts, Professor Alston came over to me.

"That was excellent, Yvonne. You showed them how to do a presentation; that's the way to do it," she said.

"Thank you, Professor. I must confess that I had previous experience," I said.

Later, when she gave us our marks, I received an A+.

During the second half of the course, we explored more vernacular traditions, including gospel, songs of social change, jazz, and rhythm and blues. We traversed to the period termed Literary Realism, Naturalism, Modernism (1940-1960). The literature published during that era was mainly urban and Northern, set in Harlem and cities like Chicago and Boston. We read *Native Son* by Richard Wright. The novel incorporated the hatred, fear, and violence that existed in the culture; however, it also set the mood for African American authors to win major book awards. Gwendolyn Brooks won a Pulitzer Prize for *Annie Allen* in 1950. Ralph Ellison's *Invisible Man*, published in 1952, won the National Book Award. The poetry published during this period challenged debate about social protests.

African Americans also produced plays during this era. Lorraine Hansberry created *A Raisin in the Sun* in 1959 and won the New York Critics Circle Award for drama. As I read that play, graphic imagery sprang to life. I visualized Mama, the matriarch of a black family living on the South Side of Chicago in the 1950s, binding her clan together with love. She was caring and determined to fulfill her ambition to own a house. Realizing that owning real estate is key to long-term progress and stability, Mama went off on her own and used money from her deceased husband's life insurance policy to purchase a house in a white neighbourhood.

Hansberry's portrayal of the reaction of the white community and the extent they undertook to stop blacks from living in "their" domain is priceless. This masterpiece has survived for decades since 1959. It is known to be the first play to portray black characters, themes, and conflicts naturally and realistically. It spawned a movie, and is still produced in theatres, even today.

We traversed to The Black Arts Era (1960-1975) and examined Dr. Martin Luther King, Jr.'s "Letter from Birmingham Jail," written in 1963. It garnered an outpouring of support for the civil rights struggle. As I read the letter, I marvelled that a person locked away in jail could have been clearheaded and focused enough to pen such a document. It was pure genius, a masterpiece in which Dr. King applied several literary devices, including allusion, anaphora, metaphors, and similes, to emphasize the white clergy's hypocrisy and lack of godliness. We also examined the autobiography of Malcolm X, published posthumously in 1965, and Amiri Baraka's play, *Dutchman*.

The course ended with contemporary literature. We examined the writings of authors, including Toni Morrison. We read Percival Everett's *Erasure*, published in 2001. It tells the story of how the publishing industry pigeonholed African American writers. The protagonist, Thelonious Monk, is a professor of English literature. He is criticized constantly for not writing *black enough*. Angered by the success of a book club's selection of a novel that reflects the stereotypical contemporary black experience, Monk created a satirical response based on Richard Wright's *Native Son*. He titled it *My Pafology,* then changed it to *Fuck*. A Hollywood producer, a talk show host, and a panel of famous novelists willingly accepted the brutal, degraded black character in the novel rather than Monk, the middle-class intellectual of Ellison's first protagonist.

If anyone wishes to learn about African American literature and its evolution without doing a course, *The Norton Anthology of African American Literature* is an excellent text to read.

By studying African American literature, I climbed to the mountaintop and reached the summit, the apex of enlightenment. I felt like one of the black intellectuals. My cup ran over.

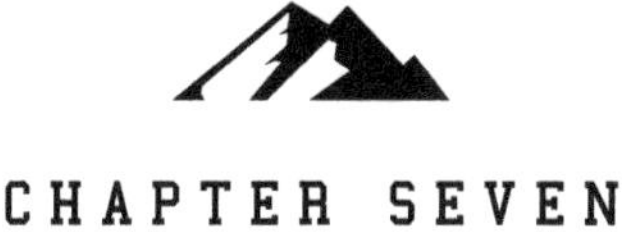

CHAPTER SEVEN

The Eccentric Professor

"When I look at my clothes, I think of them as an expression of the joy and fun of fashion—with a bit of English eccentricity thrown in."

—SUZY MENKES

My journey to York University navigated a long, circuitous road. I wanted to visit the continent of Africa, the land of my ancestors, for many years, but the media was brutal reporting on that continent. The press was always negative. The depressing news made me deliberate, dawdle, and delay the journey many times.

In the spring of 1997, my sister-in-law, who had married a Nigerian and lived in Nigeria for twenty years, visited me in Toronto. She seemed hale, healthy, and happy. The photographs of her five children portrayed them as healthy and well cared for. What had I expected? I decided then to visit Mother Africa later that year, with the plan to spend some time with my sister-in-law in Nigeria and some time in Ghana, the country I believed the ancestors of my maternal grandmother originated. I travelled alone. I can only say that the journey was very spiritual.

Returning home to Toronto, I invited several friends over for dinner. During the evening, I shared photographs I took on the journey that I had hurriedly printed and anecdotes about incidences I encountered in Africa. My guests responded with enthusiasm and insisted that I share the stories with others. “Write a book about your journey,” they said. I thought about it and thought about it and concluded that they were right; I should share my story with the world.

I had been a banker all my working life, and had never written anything for publication before, so I did everything you should do to become a writer. I read extensively about writing. Looking back, I believe I read every book in the library in the section about writing. I read books on how to write articles, short stories, and novels. I bought books about writing that I use as references even today. I attended workshops and seminars about writing, joined a writer’s group, and entered writing competitions. I wrote columns for newspapers and published short stories. In essence, I did all I could to hone my writing skill. I worked ardently for two years to produce a well-written book that was commercially viable. *Into Africa: A Personal Journey*, my first book, became a category bestseller on Amazon.com in 2002. The road was long and winding, but it was the publication of the book that led me to York U.

* * *

In May 2015, I registered for the summer course, The Short Story. The description stated it would cover the short story from its inception in the early nineteenth century to the current time and would approach it critically through the lenses of feminism, Marxism, realism, fantasy, and detective stories.

The Short Story was one of two courses I took that occurred at night, from 7:00 p.m. to 10:00 p.m. I caught the YRT bus and disembarked near the York Lanes entrance. I arrived early for the first class and selected a seat in the middle of the room. As I waited, I retrieved the course kit from my backpack and reread the first short story listed in the syllabus, "Fall of the House of Usher." At 6:45 p.m., I looked up as the professor walked into the room. For a moment, I thought I had entered a fairy tale.

You may think I'm too darn critical of people when I write about the professor of this course. I am not. I try to be open-minded about my fellow human beings until they overtly show their true colours. But I am an author, and authors are curious. We observe things, spy on things, record things, listen in on people's conversations, and use bits and pieces of the information gathered to flavour our prose stew. I'll call the professor Eva to protect the innocent. Eva was simply a suitable subject to observe and document.

Below is a transcript of the notes I wrote in my notebook on the first day of the class:

"Eva is an old woman (maybe 90) with wild platinum-blond hair scooped back into a bun at the nape of her neck, her tiny breasts hang low down, skinny. Today, she wears a green sweater, plaid skirt, leopard patterned stockings and black patent-leather loafers. Her handbag is brown leather. She wears gold wire-rim glasses."

After the other students arrived and the class began, Professor Eva informed us that she does not do email. If we wanted to get in touch with her, we should phone the English Department and leave a message with the secretary. "She must be kidding," I thought. Who would imagine a professor teaching at a prestigious institute of higher learning in the twenty-first century who did not use email? I was flabbergasted. Snickering erupted around me.

Professor Eva spoke in a voice similar to Bernadette's on *The Big Bang Theory,* making her more intriguing. She wasted no time with pleasantries and promptly laid out the format the classes would take. From 7:00 to 8:00 p.m., she would present her ideas about the text assigned for each lesson. She would allow us to ask questions and have discussions; then there would be a short break. From 8:15, students would do seminar presentations, covering any major issues we encountered in the stories we read for the class. Students must provide her with typed copies of their presentations at the beginning of each class. Professor Eva warned that she would not accept any writing done in bullet form. We must write in complete sentences in the document. Students must also include two questions for class discussion and provide their own answers.

After I recovered from the shock of Professor Eva's appearance, I concentrated on the coursework. She marched us through the syllabus methodically like a drill sergeant in the army. She allowed no deviation from the course plan. We examined short stories written by renowned authors, including Alice Munro, William Trevor, Edgar Allan Poe, and Arthur Conon Doyle, focusing on the theory of the short story.

I had written and published a few short stories, employing knowledge gained from workshops and my readings on the subject, before I began attending the class. Professor Eva burrowed deep into the theory of the short story, exposing me to aspects I had not discovered.

In the summer months, the sun is just retiring at 9:00 p.m. Professor Eva ended the classes twenty minutes early, and as I rode the bus home, darkness began to spread its gloved hand over the city. I never worried about attending classes at night. I felt safe.

By the end of the course, Professor Eva taught us that the short story is didactic, it has compactness, it has a point—an underlying value system—it has unity of effect, and it has a milieu (her favourite word). Our brains overflowed with information. We were raring and ready to write our masterpiece.

The axiom, "Don't judge a book by its cover," aptly applied to Professor Eva. Despite her odd appearance, the mismatched colours of her clothing, and her unsmiling face (I never saw her smile once), she was well versed in the genre she taught and imparted knowledge excellently. I gained valuable knowledge from the course, but it did not deter me from recording a few more of her outfits in my notebook:

June 2rd: *Professor Eva wears a pleated skirt, a blue sweater, and patterned tights.*

June 9th*: Professor Eva wore a beige top, green sweater, a houndstooth patterned skirt that stopped just below her knees, the usual black loafer with beige socks with a frilly lace top that she turned down!*

June 14th: *Today, Professor wears a beige cotton pleated skirt, a white blouse with collar, and a baby-blue sweater. She wears the same black patent-leather loafers with white socks.*

June 18th: *A different outfit today! Cream coloured blouse with collar covered partly by a red round-neck sweater. Skirt—cream background with large red patterns. Still wearing the black patent leather shoes, off-white socks with tops turned down.*

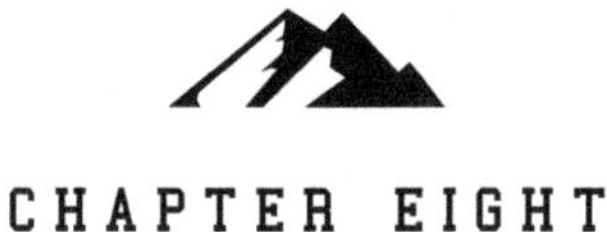

CHAPTER EIGHT

Practical Lessons for Daily Life

"You must do the things you think you cannot do."
—ELEANOR ROOSEVELT

After I'd completed a few English courses and obtained excellent grades for each, my confidence ratcheted up. I felt I could now tackle any subject and figured the time had come to explore some non-literature courses. I needed six credits in natural science for my degree, so I checked out the courses offered under that discipline. I carefully read the brief overview for Understanding Food on the university's website. It specified that the course is "A study of what food is, where it comes from and the roles various foods play in human and health nutrition." I noted it did not mention scientific formulas. Of course, that didn't mean there wouldn't be any; however, it stated that knowledge of science was not required. That statement put my mind at ease. I registered for it.

On the first day of the course, I entered the Accolade East Building, one I had never been inside before. I walked into a large lecture theatre. The seats were arranged theatre-style, at a steep angle, in three sections divided by two aisles. After several minutes, the room filled up. There must have been five hundred students present. "Whoa! This must be a popular course," I thought. Professor Monaldi was a middle-aged woman wearing glasses, slacks, and a sweater, with the body of a twenty-year-old. She stood on a platform at the front of the room, a microphone in her hand. Eight of her teaching assistants sat in the front row.

The professor introduced herself, speaking with a thick accent I could not decipher. She provided a more detailed overview of the course, and explained how the classes would operate. For assignments and grading, she divided the class into several small groups. She placed students in groups using letters of the alphabet; therefore, you had no say in selecting your group members. My group consisted of five students. Professor Monaldi asked for volunteers to act as group representatives. A student in the middle of the room stood up and asked if we had to learn any scientific formulas. The professor replied that we need not stress ourselves over formulas, but there would be a few.

After dispensing with the housekeeping items, Professor Monaldi began to lecture. She delivered two sobering statements:

"Whatever we eat, we depend on other living organisms on earth."

"There is no single food that can satisfy all our needs."

I reflected on the statements, and realized that whether we regarded ourselves as vegans, vegetarians, or omnivores, we ate other organisms.

Of all the professors I studied with at York U., Professor Monaldi was the only one I had no interaction with (until COVID-19 arrived). She remained distant and remote, standing on the stage with her microphone, moving about as she lectured, never coming near the students. Of course, I understood why—the class was too large. She did ask a few questions during lectures, and students stood at their spots and shouted their responses.

Despite the remoteness of the professor, I must say that Understanding Food proved to be the course in which I learned the most about practical things to do. I still apply some of these learnings to my daily life. But no matter how hard you try, you can't remove the "science" from natural science. We spent the first three lectures learning about the scientific attributes of foods; micro and macro molecules; micronutrients—substances that are indispensable to our bodies but needed in small amounts; and macronutrients—nutrients required in large quantities for us to survive. We studied amino acids, the most important vitamins, and what they provide, plus lipids, carbohydrates, and the importance of water in our bodies.

After that, we explored where food comes from. I learned how food is grown, and its production, processing, preservation, distribution, and enrichment. I learned about the nutritional value of food today and how it has changed over the years. For example, the broccoli we eat today has decreased in nutrients by 50 percent between 1950 and 1999.

The lecture about utensils held my interest as I absorbed information about pots and pans I had never known before: cast iron does not conduct heat very well but holds heat because of its density and thickness; stainless steel is a poor conductor of heat, but good quality stainless steel pots are sandwiched with other metals like copper that improves conduction; copper transfers heat excellently, but copper ions can enter the food, so copperware is usually lined with tin or stainless steel; aluminum cookware conducts heat well and is cheap and lightweight, but it reacts to some food substances like acid, can leach into food, and is toxic to our diets; glass dishes like Pyrex, and ceramic bowls like Corning cookware, are not good conductors of heat like metals, but they can withstand quick temperature changes and are better suited for oven or microwave cooking. Why had I not learned all these things in my twenties when I was newly married and cooking up a storm?

Professor Monaldi seemed to have a collection of profound statements that she unleashed on the class now and again.

This one had me thinking deeply: "Cooking is tied to our humanity. No other species cook!"

I cast my mind back to the animals I knew. Imagery of wolves, lions, and hyenas tearing apart raw meat and eating it came into view. I visualized our pets at home, waiting for us to feed them. It was true: no other species cook!

We explored the industrialization of food. I was astounded to discover that the production of food in the Western world is virtually controlled by six large corporations—a global oligopoly, the professor called it.

Perhaps the segment of the course that I found most interesting was about beverages. I had habitually drunk a cup of coffee each morning but had switched to tea several years ago. Professor Monaldi pointed out that coffee does not give us energy. It is not a macronutrient; however, it boosts our energy. The information about tea from the *Camellia sinensis* bush (not herbal teas) fascinated me so much that after completing the course, I researched it further. I even built a website that provided information about tea, from production to processing to consumption, to its numerous health benefits.

The professor lectured on genetics and food. I had always been leery of genetically modified organisms (GMOs) and wanted to know more. I gained better insight about them from the lectures.

Professor Monaldi gave us two quizzes, one after the fourth week, the other after the tenth week. She also gave us four group assignments that we had to do during the activity period and hand in on the same day. I was annoyed with two members of my group who did no work and left the burden of completing group assignments on the shoulders of three of us. We did our best, and our hard work paid off. We managed to obtain good grades.

Midterm arrived. The midterm exam did not take place in the lecture hall. It took place simultaneously in several rooms because of the class size. In my exam room, students sat one desk apart from each other. The tension in the room became so thick you could have chopped it with a cleaver. I must admit that I became a tad nervous. It was my first natural science course and my first natural science midterm exam. Also, much of the stuff I'd learned was new to me. I had attended all the lectures and listened attentively. I took copious notes, read the assigned texts, and reviewed all of my notes. We had covered a lot by the halfway mark. Would I remember all that I had learned? Did I reread the subjects that Professor Monaldi included in the exam?

Showtime. One of the invigilators told us to put away all textbooks and electronic devices. Only student cards, pencils, and pens were allowed on the desks. She distributed exam booklets that we were permitted to open only when instructed. The countdown clock started. I opened my booklet and observed that the exam consisted of fifty multiple-choice questions.

Multiple-choice questions! What the heck was this? In my college days, no such thing as multiple-choice exam questions existed. You either knew the answer to a question and wrote it in your own words, paying attention to your spelling and grammar, or you did not know and wrote an incorrect answer.

Realizing my time was limited to answer fifty questions, I put aside my twentieth-century thoughts, now regarded as old-school, and read the first question. Four potential answers, listed as A, B, C, and D below the question, consisted of a nuance of the answer, the opposite of the answer, an erroneous answer, and the correct answer. Any one of the answers, except the correct one, could lead you astray. You had to have read the text and remembered its exact wording to answer the questions correctly. The nuanced answer was a red herring. Although you could have guessed some answers, it would be impossible to guess enough correct ones to receive a passing grade. Okay, so multiple-choice questions were not as simple as I'd thought. It seemed that the twenty-first-century highfalutin method of testing was foolproof. I read all questions carefully, racked my aged brain, and then used my pencil to shade in the little circle at the end of each answer I selected.

On my way home, sitting on the bus, I mulled over the questions on the exam and recalled my answers. I flipped through my notes, and mentally calculated the marks I thought I would receive. I computed 94 percent. When the TA provided the results, I received 96 percent. Great Scott! My aged brain had worked perfectly. For the final exam, I received 92 percent.

Professor Monaldi concluded the course by reiterating that "Food is fundamental to the health and wellbeing of all citizens…food is a matter of national security."

* * *

In July, Ada, one of my Caribbean posse ladies, telephoned me early one morning. In the middle of my hello, she erupted into song—the Happy Birthday song. I laughed all the way through her singing. Ada didn't have the most melodious voice, but it was the thought that mattered. She remembered my birthday and took time to call.

"Oh, Ada, that was so sweet. Thank you," I said when the singing ended.

Of course, it was an annual ritual. Ada has been singing the birthday song to me every birthday for several years. It used to bother me that I forgot her birthday many times. With my improved memory, I intended to remedy that problem.

"I'm taking you out for lunch later. You choose the restaurant. Are any good ones up there in your area?"

"There's a small Middle Eastern restaurant on Yonge Street, a short distance from my home," I said.

"Sounds good; let's try it."

Ada lives in Markham, the adjoining suburb south of where I live, hence the "up there." She drove to my home, parked her car in the driveway, and insisted we walk to the restaurant. My birthday month is a time when the heat and humidity can be unbearable. That day, the weather was near perfect, the sky clear blue and cloudless, but noon was not the ideal time for walking. We arrived at the restaurant hot and dripping with sweat. Ada immediately ordered cool drinks before we examined the menu. While we waited, she looked around the room.

"There's hardly anyone here. If this is all the customers they get, they'll soon have to close," she said.

"I suspect most of their patrons are Middle Eastern who are probably more into eating out at dinnertime," I said.

We ate slowly, savouring the spicy *koftas* we'd ordered, feeling as though we had the restaurant to ourselves. My mind floated back to Understanding Food, the course I'd recently completed, and the lessons I'd learned about where food comes from and the various ways of cooking it. I wondered what method the chef of the restaurant had used. We discussed the issues of the day and the past.

Suddenly, Ada said, "My goodness, Yvonne, your memory is so good now. I can't believe you remember all those things."

We both laughed at the irony of the situation. I used to be the one who would forget most things while Ada would remind me of them. The tables had turned.

"You know something, Ada, studying at the university and using my brain cells regularly has helped immensely. I'm surprised at how much more I remember now. You should sign up for even a few courses."

Ada held fast that although studying seemed great for my memory, she was unwilling to try it.

"Girl, I admire you for your determination, but I couldn't do it. Bless your heart."

We spent an hour and a half in the restaurant, then walked back to my home. I appreciated the walk that time. The extra calories we had eaten needed a match to set them on fire.

CHAPTER NINE

Strive for Better

"Be so good they can't ignore you."
—STEVE MARTIN

The motto of the International Olympic Committee (IOC) is "Faster, Higher, Stronger." These are the goals Olympians strive to achieve. As a senior citizen and certainly not an Olympian, I did not aim for superlatives; however, I never wanted to be a mediocre student receiving just passing grades at York U. From the beginning, I'd set a benchmark that my grade on each subject should be a minimum of a B. If I received a higher grade, I would be overjoyed; however, any grade below a B would not be satisfactory for my efforts. I knew that earning good grades meant doing the work. In my case, extra effort was required since retention was not as easy as it was in my college days. To this end, I utilized my time wisely.

There are dozens of nooks, crannies, and cozy spots at York U. where you could park your derriere, pull out your textbooks, and study. I preferred to study at home; however, some days, I had to remain on campus for another class, and I refused to waste time. While some of my younger peers sprawled everywhere, sitting on the floor, on stairs, and leaning against walls, I dashed into The Sound and Moving Image Library. I would have had difficulty getting up if I'd sat on the floor; I knew my limitations. I found the TSMI library to be a quiet, comfortable hideaway. Located on the main floor of the Scott Library, it housed a multidisciplinary media collection available to the York University community for educational, research, and personal use. Of course, I did not use this library for research. The high-ceilinged room where you check out material has several cubicles separated individually. Here you could plug your ear with earbuds and watch movies on computers. I spent many hours between classes in one of those cubicles, reading textbooks and writing assignments. It was easy to dash out for my classes.

* * *

York U. is an active community, and students participate in numerous activities outside of their academic studies. Clubs abound on campus, including religious and social ones. Walking through Vari Hall into the wide hallway of the Ross Building, you will frequently see tables manned by students and arranged with posters and brochures advertising one event or another. Sometimes students sell cookies or muffins to raise funds.

York U.'s football team, called The Lions, has existed since 1968 and represents the university in Ontario in Canadian football and University Sports. The team has never won a championship, yet the fans remain enthusiastic year after year.

I did not get involved in any ongoing university extracurricular activities, not because I didn't want to, but because I didn't have the time. Although I was a student, my regular life continued as before. My time was at a premium; however, I participated in the annual voting for members of the Student Council of Liberal Arts and Professional Studies (SCOLAPS). The candidates usually advertised heavily, with posters pasted on walls everywhere and advertisements in the university's newspaper. Sometimes they solicited students walking through Vari Hall and the Ross Building. I also occasionally attended the Speaker Series talks. If speakers planned to discuss topics that interested me, I remained after class and attended.

Participation in extracurricular activities is a positive and valued thing in the university community. Some scholarship application forms listed community involvement as a requirement to qualify for scholarships, plus good grades.

* * *

As my studies continued, I expended great effort to maintain contact with friends. I had accumulated an array of friends from several ethnic groups after I had worked thirty-seven years in the banking industry, sat on several boards, sat on federal, provincial, and Municipal government committees, served as a volunteer for many years, and travelled around the world. A funny thing happened: I observed a change in the attitude of only some of my black friends. I became the person who did most of the telephoning. Responses included excuses like, "I didn't call because I know you're busy with your studies" or "I know you're swamped with schoolwork, so I didn't want to bother you." The explanations they gave for not calling aroused my curiosity. I had never told anyone that I was swamped with schoolwork. Why did they assume that? I will acknowledge that I became hard-pressed a few times to complete and deliver assignments on time; however, those were fleeting moments that I would never allow to disrupt friendships. Spending a minute or two on a phone call wouldn't be detrimental to my studies. My primary activity outside of class time, and one reason for retiring early, had been to write. I spent many hours writing each week.

My studies progressed satisfactorily and were on track until a strike occurred at York U. Members of the Canadian Union of Public Employees, who worked for the university, walked off their jobs in

March 2015. York U. cancelled all classes because union membership included contract faculty who taught classes and hundreds of teaching and graduate assistants who ran tutorials and labs and marked papers. Although almost a thousand members of the union ratified a deal soon after, the university remained closed. Students were back in their classes after a month. I did not register for a summer course that year, which added a semester or two to the time I had planned to complete my degree.

* * *

The Holy Land had been an important place on my bucket list to visit. I'd put off going there several times, mainly because I wanted to visit Egypt on the same trip. In July 2013, the army overthrew President Morsi of Egypt, and killed hundreds of people. In May 2014, the former army chief Abdel Fattah al-Sisi won the presidential election. By November, the Sinai-based armed group Ansar Beyt al-Maqdis pledged allegiance to the extreme Islamic State movement, which controls parts of Syria and Iraq. The situation became more and more dangerous in Egypt. I struck it off my list.

In the autumn of 2015, I completed a Bible study called Walking Where Jesus Walked. In addition to the text, the facilitator showed videos highlighting several places in the Holy Land. It rekindled my desire to go on the journey. Two months later, by sheer coincidence (or was it divine intervention?), Natalie, my best friend from high school, phoned me from Boston to say that her sister's church in New York City planned to go on a tour of the Holy Land in the New Year, and she intended to go. Would I join the group? I would not miss the opportunity for the world, I told her. Natalie emailed me the details of the tour with an impressive itinerary. I signed up immediately. I asked Gloria, one of my Caribbean posse ladies, to accompany me, and she agreed. We flew to New York and overnighted at the Holiday Inn near JFK airport. The next morning, we joined the rest of the tour group at the airport. On the 4th of January, 2016, we flew to the Holy Land.

I had already registered for a winter course to begin the first week in January. Going on the trip meant I would miss the first two classes. From my observation, the first class involved mainly introductions, discussions about syllabuses, and explanations of how classes would operate. Professors rarely taught a lesson. I would merely have to obtain notes on the second class from a classmate. With that in mind, I put my studies on the back burner and placed my mind in gear to enjoy the Holy Land.

The tour delivered much more than I'd anticipated. We sailed up the Sea of Galilee (a lake really), visited Mt. Beatitude—the place where Jesus taught the Beatitudes, and also the Church of the Primacy of St. Peter at Tabgha, where Mensa Christi, a large limestone rock, sits inside. It is said to be the spot where Jesus served his disciples bread and fish after his resurrection. We visited Capernaum, Megiddo, where we viewed the Jezreel Valley mentioned in the book of Revelation and said to be the area where Armageddon will be fought. We also visited Caesarea, the River Jordan, Qumran, the place where Bedouin shepherds found the Dead Sea Scrolls, Jericho, the Dead Sea, Nazareth, Bethlehem, and of course, the city of Jerusalem. I took a side trip to visit Masada. There, I saw the incredible ruins of the fortress that King Herod built atop a mountain that overlooks the Judean wilderness and the Dead Sea.

Despite the limited times available for travelling while attending York U., and not wanting to travel in the summer when the weather is good in Toronto, I managed to tour Turkey, three Hawaiian Islands—the Big Island, Maui, and O'ahu—Barbados, and Jamaica.

At the end of my second year at York U., I reread the Academic Calendar for the Faculty of Liberal Arts & Professional Studies and made an appointment to meet with a guidance counsellor for the English department. Why? I wanted to make sure that my studies remained on track and that I did not waste time taking courses that would not contribute to the degree. I sat before the counsellor at his desk, and he pulled up my record on his computer. Gazing at the screen, he exclaimed, "You are doing so well! You should consider going to grad school when you complete the degree." I thanked him for the compliment but assured him that attending grad school did not interest me. He painstakingly reviewed the English program checklist he had printed in preparation for our meeting. He used a highlighter to mark the courses I had done and the areas I still had to complete. I made similar appointments every subsequent year. The counsellors always suggested that I attend grad school.

As I progressed through the courses, I observed that several of my young classmates seemed to put little effort into their studies. What were they thinking? Were they so brilliant that they did not need to make any effort? In one instance, halfway through a semester, one classmate piped up that he did not have the textbook for the course. He was not willing to purchase it and had been on the waiting list to borrow it from the library, but it had not become available. I usually purchased my textbooks at least a week before each class began, provided the university bookstore had them in stock. I bought some books via Amazon a few times to have them in time for class. I usually read the text early to be prepared for class discussions.

One day, at the end of a Modern Canadian Fiction class, Professor Winter, a short man with curly hair, wearing glasses with thick lenses, reminded us to read *The Double Hook* for discussion in the next class. We were to apply "close reading" by considering style (motifs and their meaning), settings, and imagery. We had ample warning and time to read the novel since the date to discuss it was in the syllabus from the first lesson.

Fourteen students attended the next class. After Professor Winter gave his usual hour-long lecture, we had a break; then the time came to discuss *The Double Hook*. I was the only student who had completed the reading. No discussion occurred that day. The reading materials for Modern Canadian Fiction consisted of eleven novels and a short story collection. I read them all. How many of these books would my classmates read? I wondered about the grades they would receive at the end of the course. Did they think cramming the night before the midterm and final exams would earn them good grades? Professors allotted a certain percentage of the overall marks for participation in every class, sometimes as much as 10 percent.

Why forfeit marks for participation and rely solely on exam results? I couldn't fathom the behaviour of my classmates.

During the second semester of the course, Professor Winter gave us the assignment to write our final essay. We were to write a research essay comparing two novels we had read. I searched databases online for hours via my York U. account, trying to find at least two academic papers that supported my thesis. The articles from JSTOR always provided the best information for my research essays. JSTOR did not disappoint. I tended to over-research for my assignments and found five excellent articles. Having too much information could be as bad as having too little, so I narrowed it down to the two that best supported my argument. I submitted my essay, and felt confident that I'd done a great job.

Two months after the course ended, I received the email below from Professor Winter:

> a@yorku.ca
> To: Blackwood
>
> *Yvonne:*
> *Hi! How's your summer going?*
> *I would like to nominate your final essay for an essay prize, particularly the Avie Bennett Prize in Canadian literature. While it's past the official deadline, I've been given an extension (like so many students...) The copy I have is the one that you submitted to Turnitin. Do you have a title for the essay? I don't recall if you had one on the hard copy. Please let me know as soon as you can. No big deal if you don't have one.*
> *Thanks, A.W.*

The email blew me away. Had I mastered the art of essay writing? Was my work good enough to be entered into a competition? I replied immediately and told the professor to go ahead and submit the essay.

In November, I received a letter from the English Department. It stated in part that:

> *"While the adjudicators were impressed both by the sophistication and elegance of your essay, your application was not the successful one. The committee very much hopes that you have another opportunity to apply again at the end of the current academic year."*

I sent Professor Winter this email:

> <blackwood>:
> *Hello Professor Winter, I hope you are having a good time. I don't know if the English Department contacted you regarding the essay you submitted. I've just received this letter from the department, and I thought I would share it with you. Although I did not win, I want to thank you wholeheartedly for submitting the essay. It certainly gives me a boost to strive for excellence.*
> *I know you are away from school, but probably checking your email.*
> *Much regards,*
> *Yvonne Blackwood*

Professor Winter replied:

> a@yorku.ca
> To: Blackwood
>
> Nov. 12,
> *Hi. Yes, I did get this (and yes, I check my email all the time). I'm disappointed, but the fact is that it's an excellent essay and I can tell you from having sat*

> *on the committee that judges these things that the competition is fierce. Sometimes it comes down to a very close vote. You're a fine student, and I was very happy to have you in my class!*
> *All best wishes on your future studies and other endeavours!*
> *A.W.*

By the middle of the third year, my conscientious, disciplined work, paid off. One evening at home in August, scanning through my emails, I noticed one from York University. I opened it and read:

> *"As a result of your outstanding academic results in the Summer 2016 session and/or the Fall/Winter 2016-2017 academic sessions, you have been awarded the York University Continuing Student Scholarship. The scholarship has been applied directly to your online student account...."*

At first, I thought of deleting the email, thinking it must be a scam or a prank. It contained the logo of the university, but I knew that scammers are good at replicating logos. I reread the email, then signed into my student account. The scholarship funds rested in the account. The email was authentic. I was shocked. First, I hadn't applied for any scholarships. Second, I didn't think that the university gave scholarships to mature students. Third, I was not aware that anyone had been tracking my grades. Once I recovered from the surprise, I read about how to thank donors and tried to comply.

A couple of weeks later, I received a letter from The Golden Key International Honour Society requesting that I become a member. I had never heard of them before. I read the brochure that accompanied the letter, then researched the organization on the Internet. The society was legitimate and had existed since 1977. It is devoted to helping its members achieve excellence through the advancement of academics, leadership, and service. It has more than two million members worldwide and chapters in several countries and offers membership to university students from around the world but only to high-achieving students in the top 15 percent of their programs. Golden Key provides scholarships to students and conducts seminars and summits. York U. is one of its member universities. I appreciated the offer but thought, "I'm an old retiree who has lived a full life. Let all their offerings go to the younger students who need it more than I."

I threw out the letter.

The powers that be placed my name on the Dean's List. Later, I received an invitation to a breakfast for the top undergraduate students. It stated:

> *"Your name was selected from a list of York students who have displayed a strong academic performance. The Dean of the Faculty of Graduate Studies would like to welcome you to a morning reception to celebrate your achievements and tell you a little about graduate education at York."*

I was flattered to the tenth degree. Sure, I had worked hard and received excellent grades beyond my goal; however, I had not anticipated this much success. At the beginning of this story, I mentioned that my goal was to obtain a bachelor's degree in English to help me to add texture to my writing. I had no plan or desire to pursue graduate studies. I did not attend the breakfast. Every subsequent year, I received letters from York U. advising me to apply for scholarships.

The Golden Key International Honour Society persisted. After receiving two more letters asking me to join the society, I completed the application form and paid the one-time membership fee. In May 2019, I attended a Golden Key reception held at York University's Founders Assembly Hall. The president of York U.'s chapter and three interesting guests delivered speeches. I walked across the stage and received my membership certificate.

It was written in beautiful Old English style and stated:

> This Certifies that Mrs. Yvonne Blackwood in Recognition of Outstanding Scholastic Achievement and Excellence has been granted membership in Golden Key International Honour Society and is herby granted all the Rights, Honours and Privileges pertaining to the Society at York University.

I was pleased to see several students there, indicating they had also obtained excellent grades. I couldn't help but notice that I was the oldest student present.

The scholarship from the university and the Golden Key membership boosted my resolve to pursue my studies. *Tentanda via.* I was finding a way as I continued to climb the mountain. Glimpses of the summit were beginning to appear through the mist. I now aimed to earn As instead of Bs. York U. remained supportive of my efforts and awarded me continuing student scholarships in 2018 and 2019.

CHAPTER TEN

A Pressure Cooker

"Our limitations and success will be based, most often, on your own expectations for ourselves. What the mind dwells upon, the body acts upon."

—DENIS WAITLEY

Summer courses are hard. They are hard because they are compressed. A three-credit course is usually taught over a semester; a six-credit course extends over two semesters. The length of summer courses is cut in half, while the course instructions remain the same. It goes without saying that you have to work twice as hard and twice as fast to complete the work in half the time. I experienced the accelerated pace when I took The Short Story in the summer of 2015, but that was a three-credit course.

In 2016, I registered for my first humanities course, knowing I must obtain nine credits in that discipline to earn my degree. Exuding confidence, I ventured to take a six-credit summer course. While perusing the humanities course directory, I read the titles of all the courses offered that year and realized the discipline was all-encompassing. The Bible in Modern Context caught my attention. How difficult could a course about the Bible be? I grew up in the church, attended Sunday school from age four, and attended church every Sunday to age eighteen. I'd memorized numerous Bible verses during my youth; some I remember to this day. I had accepted Christ later in life and attended church regularly. I had served my church as the head usher and was presently the head teller. Thinking about all my church teachings and activities, I signed up for the course, convinced it would be a cinch.

Classes took place in Calumet College, one of the farthest buildings on campus from the bus stop where I got off. To get there, I had to walk across two fields, descend a steep hill, pass the Norman Bethune building, and cross a narrow bridge. On the first day, I arrived at the classroom assigned to the course and found it in disarray. Desks and chairs were scattered about the room as though students had engaged in a fight. "This is not a good sign for a religious course," I thought. It was probably a sign that the course would be rocky, but I didn't know it then. Two male students entered the room immediately after me. We looked questioningly at each other, then worked diligently to put the room in order. The starting time for the class was 4:00 p.m.

Professor Damian, a short man of about sixty with grey hair, bald in the centre of his head and with a conspicuous birthmark at the front left side, arrived ten minutes before start time. He was clean-shaven and wore a short-sleeve plaid shirt, dark pants, and sandals. I smiled when I saw the sandals—Jesus shoes, I thought. He quickly set up the computer in the room and distributed copies of the syllabus to the thirty students who had arrived. And right there on the first page of the syllabus, under the words "course description," was a sentence that gave me cause to pause:

"Students who have concluded that the Bible is a divine revelation of God's will, and as such, is without error, may not enjoy this course and are urged to think long and hard about whether or not they wish to subject their religious faith to rational academic inquiry."

What was it saying? Was it saying that the course might corrupt a

Christian person? What could this man with a birthmark at the front left side of his head teach me in twelve weeks that would shake the belief instilled in me over sixty years? Knowing I had strong faith, I prepared my mind to hear what his words of wisdom, his "rational academic inquiry," would impart.

Professor Damian began his first lecture by saying, "We are in a class, NOT a church, or a synagogue, or a mosque, or a Hindu temple, or a Sikh gurdwara. We are here to learn perspectives, analysis, and arguments."

The students looked around at one another. One male student wore a yarmulke on his head, and two female students wore hijabs. It seemed that the class consisted of students subscribing to various religions. Professor Damian had set the stage for learning. I suspected he meant the statement as a warning that he would not tolerate anyone arguing with him, a situation he might have experienced before. He plunged into the overview of the course and emphasized that the first half would focus on the Old Testament, the second half on the New Testament. He placed a slide on the overhead. It included a timeline from 2000 BCE moving forward to 2000 CE. At that moment, I realized I had been naïve and had not paid enough attention to the course title. I had been dazzled by the words "The Bible," and overlooked the last three words, "in Modern Context," which indicated that the course would encompass history. How could one compare modern times without historical times?

Professor Damian stated that we would explore the three worlds of the Bible—the historical, the literary, and the contemporary. The historical would investigate the world behind the text and evidence outside of it to learn who wrote it, when they wrote it, to whom they wrote it, why they wrote it, and what it means in modern times. The contemporary world is the world in front of the text, what we bring to it, and what it means to us today. I was a student majoring in English and looked forward to learning about the literary aspects, especially when he hinted that the Bible contained "a lot of constructed things."

After the first lecture, the classes became like a semi racing down a steep hill without brakes. The pace moved so rapidly I had little time to do anything other than to read the texts and write assignments I had to deliver at the beginning of every class.

As we examined the Old Testament, I learned that the Jewish Bible, called the Tanakh, has twenty-four books, the Christian Bible has thirty-nine, and the first four books—common to both Bibles—is the Jewish Torah. I also learned that the Old Testament was originally written in Hebrew and date back to 1000 BCE, and that the Bible—as we know it today—was first produced in 1555.

We delved into Genesis, Exodus, and many of the books of the Old Testament, including Malachi, the last book. We kept our focus on the three worlds mentioned earlier. Professor Damian did not post his lectures on the university's website, only lecture guidelines that lacked details but were downloadable. I took notes as he spoke and wrote like the "moving finger" to capture the salient points. We viewed the film *Wall-E*, a fascinating little Disney movie. He claimed that the film really depicts the creation story in contemporary times. I had to think deeply to grasp that interpretation.

By mid-June, we arrived at the end of the study of the Old Testament and prepared to write our midterm test. I felt frayed, frazzled, and worn out.

"Oh, Lord, how much of this pressure can I take?"

I thought of quitting then and there. But how could I withdraw from the course now? I had spent an inordinate amount of energy and time reading many chapters of the *New Oxford Annotated Bible* (NOAB), plus several academic papers. I had already submitted ten assignments and written three tests. The midterm would be the fourth test. How could I throw away all of my efforts? I resorted to the two things that always calmed me down and provided a new, brighter perspective. I prayed and recited my go-to Bible verses: "Trust in the Lord with all thine heart and lean not unto thine own understanding. In all thy ways acknowledge him, and he shall direct thy paths." I found it ironic that I had to pray and read Bible verses to calm myself down while I studied the Bible. After that, I wrote the in-class test that garnered 20 percent of my mark. I left the classroom feeling that I had done a great job. The grade I received proved me correct.

* * *

The second half of the course focused on the New Testament. Knowing that it covers Christianity as we know it now, I kept the warning Professor Damian had stated in the course description in the back of my mind, and my ears pricked. He said some statements contrary to my beliefs; I took them with a drink of water from the Dead Sea.

We were engrossed in the Gospel of Mathew when the professor declared, "The Bible, and by that, I mean the Christian Bible, which includes the Old and New Testament, is one of the most widely read and most fascinating books ever written. So intriguing is this book, many scholars regard some of its prose as sublime literature."

Wait a minute, had I not heard the sublimity argument before? Yes, we had explored it in Literary Theory 1.

In one of the classes, Professor Damian had us juxtapose passages from the Gospels of Mathew, Mark, and Luke. It was riveting to observe that these texts contained some verbatim sentences, although they were written many years apart by different authors living in separate countries who were not eyewitnesses. Research showed that Mark, the first author, wrote his text in 70 CE, about forty years after the death of Jesus. Who copied who? Or was it divine intervention? We also observed the intertextuality of Old Testament text that is repeated verbatim in parts of the New Testament.

The day after we performed the juxtaposition exercise, the cool, calm, collected Professor Damian breezed into the classroom like a tornado, yelling, "Plagiarism! Plagiarism!" I had never seen him so excited, and I never saw him that way again. I thought he had caught a student who had plagiarized another person's work in one of the assignments. The professor had included the usual warning about academic integrity in his syllabus document. Who had been so stupid as to plagiarize? He promptly placed a slide on the overhead with the juxtaposed speeches by first ladies Michelle Obama and Melania Trump, given to the American people. The American media had been in an uproar that Melania Trump had plagiarized Michelle Obama's speech that she gave eight years earlier. The class read both speeches on the overhead. We never doubted for a minute that Melania Trump, even having changed a few words, had plagiarized Michelle Obama's speech.

We spent some time studying the four Gospels and highlighted their differences. Focused intently on the aspect of the literary world, I observed that the Gospel of Mark is a work that employs literary devices like metaphors, parallelism, and analogies. We examined the thirteen books attributed to the letters written by Paul the Apostle, starting with Romans. The professor claimed that six of the letters, Ephesians, Colossians, 2 Thessalonians, 1 and 2 Timothy, and Titus, were disputed as not written by Paul.

The course ended with the book of Revelation. *The New Oxford Annotated Bible with Apocrypha,* the primary textbook for the course, emphasized that "It was not written to frighten readers. It was written to bring comfort to and hope to believers who felt alienated from the synagogue and were persecuted by the Romans." The text of Revelation employs several metaphors to disguise any negative reference to the Roman Emperor.

I must say that Professor Damian taught the course well. He covered many books of the Bible in-depth and opened my eyes to many biblical incidents. I completed the course more enlightened than when I started. Although he taught the class well, he was the epitome of a slave driver. We bolted through the lessons like a bullet train heading toward its destination. Students were never allowed any room to breathe. Every class I attended (twice per week), I handed in an assignment. During the twelve-week course, I submitted twenty-one assignments and wrote six exams—one after every few classes. The pace was so hectic I thought of dropping the class more than once, but time could not douse the fires of learning in me, even with my healthy dose of old age. I stuck to my creed, "Perseverance is a great element of success…," and kept going. I needed the six credits the course offered. The time allotted to earn my degree would have increased by two semesters without those credits.

I had expected The Bible in Modern Context to be easy. It became the most stressful course I took during the entire degree program. I have no regret doing this course; however, and now apply the historical context to scripture when I read it. It makes the text more meaningful.

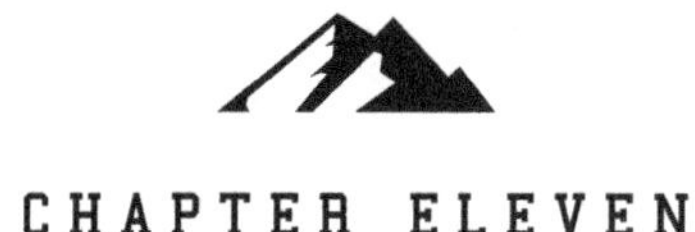

CHAPTER ELEVEN

Kindness to Fellow Faculty Member

"Human kindness has never weakened the stamina or softened the fiber of a free people."

—FRANKLIN D. ROOSEVELT

Winters can be harsh in Toronto, and by extension, they can be harsh on the extensive York U. campus grounds. The winter of 2017 included a mixture of precipitation, including mild snowfalls, blizzard-like weather, ice rain, and regular rain. The previous fall, I had registered for Modern Canadian Fiction, an English course with the objective to teach us about the development of Canadian fiction from the 1940s onward, placing that development in its historical and cultural contexts. The extensive reading list included several books by Canadian authors that I would not have otherwise read. The books included *Obasan*, *Funny Boy*, *The Double Hook*, and *The Apprenticeship of Duddy Kravitz*.

It was a six-credit course that extended over the fall and winter semesters. We were proceeding through the winter semester. I walked a long distance from Steeles Avenue to my classes in the Founders College building, though it was the closest building to the bus stop where I exited. At the end of the third lecture in January, Professor Winter announced he was changing our classroom. We were to move classes to the Norman Bethune College building for the remainder of the semester. Before that point, the university seemed to have arranged classrooms without hiccups. We started and ended classes in the same classroom. What the heck was going on? What had prompted this change? Professor Winter, our bespectacled, soft-spoken teacher, explained that the persistent bad weather had caused difficulty for a disabled professor to reach her classroom in the Norman Bethune building. He had volunteered to switch classrooms with that professor. How very noble of Professor Winter, I thought. If only there were more unselfish people like him. What I didn't know was, the danger the disabled professor experienced would be transferred to me to some degree.

On the first day of class in the Norman Bethune building, precipitation began with a mild snowfall; however, when I arrived on the campus for my class at 4:00 p.m., the snow had changed to ice rain. I'd dressed appropriately in a thick winter coat, toque, scarf, gloves, and warm insulated boots with good treads on the soles. I soon learned that good threads on soles of boots were no match for ice rain, like the brakes on a car were no match for ice on the road.

I exited the bus at the Founders Road bus stop, crossed Steeles Avenue, and entered the campus. I trekked gingerly across a field covered in ice that looked like a skating rink. Luckily, the area was flat, and although I skidded a few times, I managed to stay on my feet. I entered the Founders College building from a back door and walked indoors to the front entrance, where I exited the building and walked across a small field. I crossed a small courtyard with built-in benches where students usually gathered in the summertime. Two bronze statues depicting identical professors of the old days, dressed in trench coats and fedoras and carrying briefcases, stood in the middle of the courtyard. The bronzed professors faced each other and seemed to be enjoying a chat. The statues were usually shiny, but now they glistened with a coat of ice rain. I laughed out loud as I thought about our contemporary professors. Christ! You couldn't even tell most of them from the students. Fedoras and leather briefcases? No professor wore felt hats. Most wore jeans or corduroys, and lugged backpacks on their backs like the students. I walked by several buildings and stayed on the covered concrete walkways to avoid the ice.

The Norman Bethune building stood at the bottom of a steep hill, about one mile from where I got off the bus. I looked down the hill toward the building. The path was a glossy sheet of ice. Images flashed through my mind like the countdown at the beginning of a movie: I'm falling, falling, falling. I've broken my hip, leg, and arm. I'm in bed in a room with pristine white walls, surrounded by nurses in starched white uniforms. Oh, no! My journey to obtain an English degree has ended.

After that vivid vision, I thought of turning around and returning home. Would I be safer retracing my steps? If I did, I would have to wait at least thirty minutes, standing at a cold bus stop with the wind ripping through my coat. I reconsidered and focused on walking down the hill. I pulled myself together, mustered up every ounce of courage possible, and skirted the path, staying close to the buildings that lined the left side, praying all along that I would not fall. Somehow, I made it to the classroom without incident. During the lecture, I compelled myself not to think about the return trek back up the hill at the end of the class.

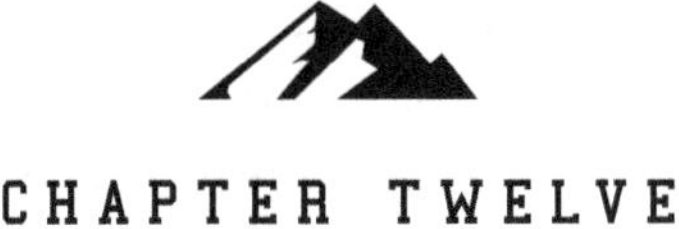

CHAPTER TWELVE

Flora, Fauna, and the Seasons

"No matter how few possessions you own or how little money you have, loving wildlife and nature will make you rich beyond measure."

—PAUL OXTON

The older I become, the more I love flora and fauna. I believe it has a lot to do with my childhood. I was raised by maternal grandparents in Manchester, a rural part of Jamaica, from age two and a half after my mother died. They were farmers, not big-time farmers with farmhands and a big farmhouse, but small subsistence farmers. They earned enough to pay the taxes on the land and feed and clothe themselves and the grandchildren they cared for. Nothing remained in the kitty to purchase luxury items, but we were happy. The old homestead, perched atop a hill, was surrounded by several acres of land, the main asset they possessed.

My grandfather cultivated one parcel of the land, opposite

the kitchen, with coffee plants interspersed with a few tangerine, grapefruit, and avocado trees. We called it "the coffee walk." The trees clustered closely together, making it dark beneath the canopy, even in the daytime. When it rained, it took some time for the water to hit the ground. Grandfather grew a large grove of ortanique trees in another section of the land. The ortanique and coffee plants bloomed tiny white flowers during the budding season, and their perfume permeated the entire yard. Oh, how I loved to smell the sweet aroma of those tiny white flowers.

As a child, I had the special chore of tending the flower garden. The garden stood immediately in front of the house and was divided into four sections, demarcated by smooth pumpkin-sized stones. My brother and I whitewashed the stones every Easter and Christmastime. In one section of the garden, we planted lilies of various species. I vividly remember the candy lilies with red and white striped, bell-shaped flowers. At a particular time of the year, not long after the blooms appeared, an army of caterpillars would descend on the plants and eat all the succulent green leaves. Nature had to take its course, I suppose. In another garden square, we grew gerberas of many colours. They would spread, and I had to divide and replant them each year. Roses populated the third section. Red roses, pink roses, white roses, and peach-coloured roses all grew together, some climbing plants, some dwarf plants. In the fourth quadrant, we cultivated a mishmash of several species of flowers—hibiscus, gladiolas, carnations, dahlias, geraniums, and more. The garden provided a paradise for hummingbirds. They frequently came, darting from one flower to another, inserting their long beaks into the blooms to extract nectar. The garden, with its whitewashed stones and the red earth packed around the roots of the plants, always boasted flowers of one kind or another that bloomed throughout the year. Every Saturday, house-cleaning day, I proudly placed a vase of fresh flowers on the high table in the hall. Now that my knees are stiff with arthritis and gardening has been curtailed, is it any wonder I love to admire plants, flowers, and animals?

* * *

During the years I travelled to and from York U., I watched the seasons change, felt the temperature shift from hot to cool to cold, and observed the plants and animals on the grounds. The campus encompassed one square kilometre of land—a vast expanse. The property had everything students would desire to be one with nature. Besides the cozy nooks and crannies indoors, there were charming enclaves outdoors that you could commandeer to relax. You could lie on the verdant manicured grass or sit under a shade tree in summer; you could watch the leaves change colour or collect pine cones in fall; you could take walks and plod through the snow that covers most of the open spaces in winter.

The university, now more than fifty years old, has grounds populated with mature trees—oak, birch, maple, and others. The most common trees are pine, their old trunks gnarled, knobby, and grey. Wherever there was a cluster of pine trees, you found pine cones covering the ground. One fall, I gathered enough dried pine cones from a single area to fill a shopping bag. I took them home and threw them into my firepit when some friends came for a barbecue. They produced a great flame and added a sweet aroma to the air.

My walking route to classes remained constant after the York Region Transit buses were no longer allowed on campus. I exited the bus at Steeles Avenue, crossed the road at the stoplights at Founders Road, and walked along a narrow-paved walkway. A network of roads crisscrossed the grounds, several designated one-way. Red triangle yield signs and black arrows direct the drivers of trucks, buses, and cars on which way to go. I crossed one of the one-way roads onto a field. At the end, I crossed another one-way road, then walked several metres to the back door of the Founders College building.

One spring morning, the air was cool and crisp as I walked across the field, heading to class. A flock of about thirty Canada geese, large and small, waddled all around me. They honked and frolicked in the grass. I crossed the second one-way road, and the geese started to cross the road too. They took their time crossing. Some even went back onto the field, then returned to the road. In the meantime, a long queue of traffic backed up as drivers waited for the geese to complete the crossing. Standing on the other side of the road, I watched the spectacle and took photos. The drivers looked frustrated, but they dared not honk their horns and confuse the geese, which would lengthen the crossing time, and they dared not run over any of them. The Canada geese are a protected species. The drivers just had to cultivate patience.

The summer my class was held in the Calumet College building, I had to descend the steep hill that leads to the Norman Bethune building. At the right side, a low concrete wall separated the path from a shallow gully. Erosion had taken place in it, and a chaos of exposed roots of the trees growing there glared up at you. The gully became a haven for fauna, and I saw several squirrels dashing up and down the trees.

A black squirrel sat on the concrete wall, holding a piece of bread with its two front feet. It nibbled the bread, looked up at passersby, and continued eating. I suspected a student had given it the bread. Further down the hill, on the left, a grey squirrel ran up to a female student and took a piece of donut she offered straight from her hand. The squirrels did not appear to mind humans at all. They had become a part of the campus landscape; it was their territory too.

Fall was my favourite season on campus. The changing colours of the leaves run the gamut from yellow to orange, to red, to brown. The maple trees displayed a spectacular show of colours. With the summer heat gone and cooler temperatures in play, you merely had to walk about the grounds and snap pictures.

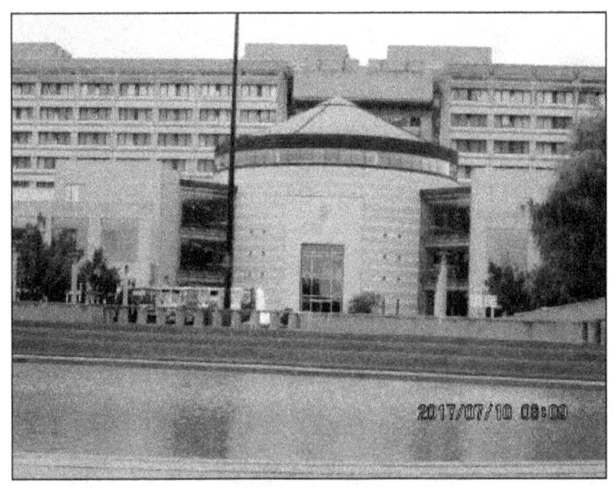

VARI HALL

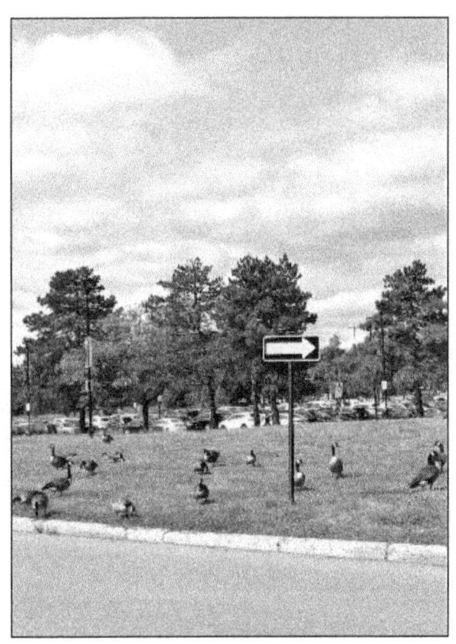

CANADA GEESE ON CAMPUS

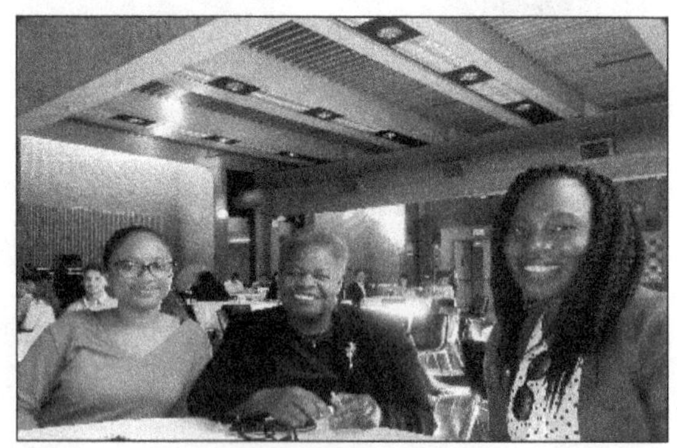

CELEBRATING GOLDEN KEY MEMBERSHIP

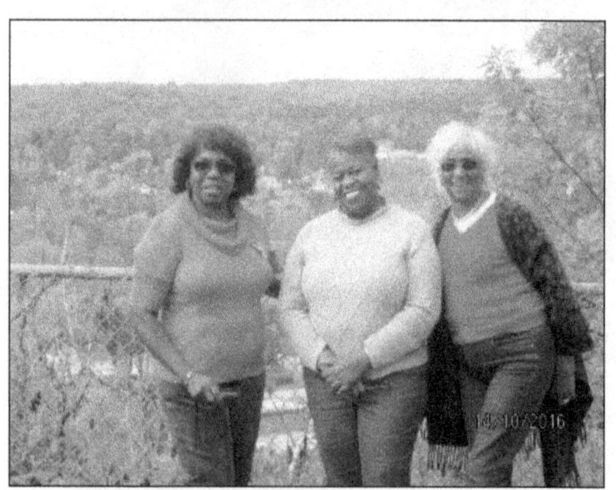

ENJOYING A FALL ROAD TRIP

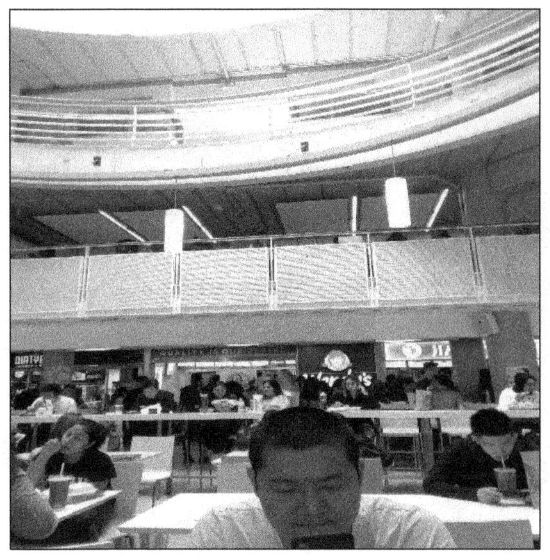

LUNCH AT FOODCOURT

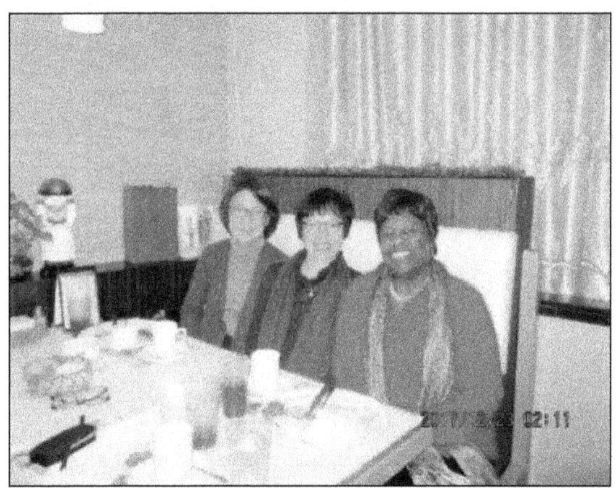

MY CHINESE POSSE

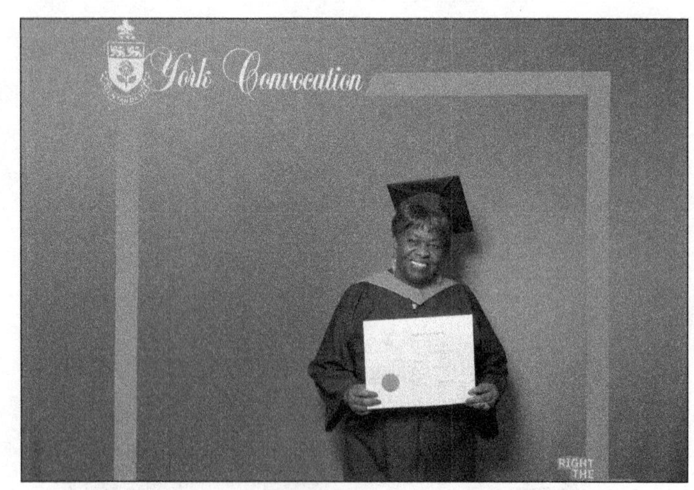

THE GRADUATE

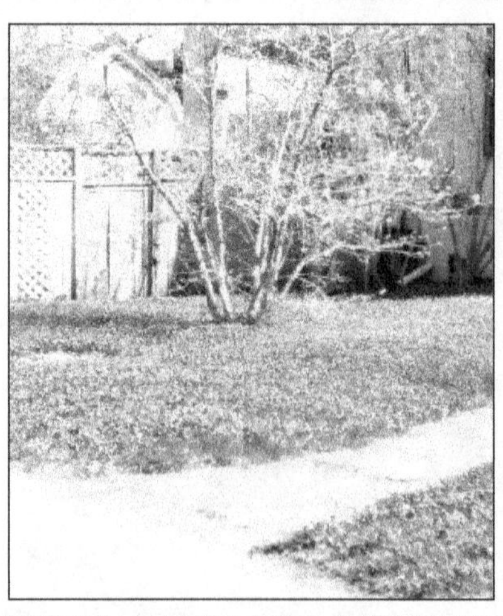

SCILLA SIBERICA TAKES OVER LAWN IN ROSEDALE

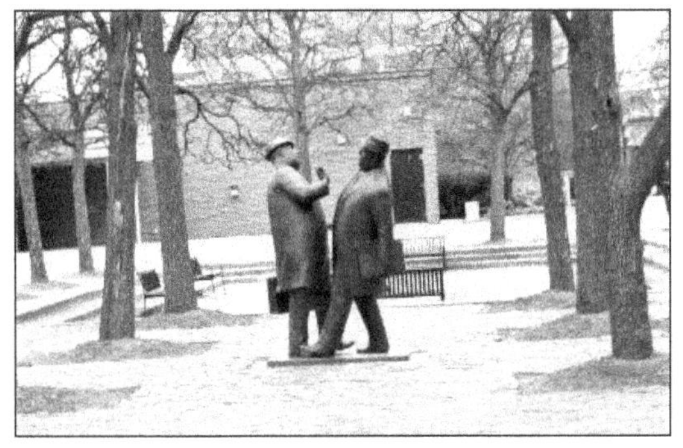

STATUE OF PROFESSORS

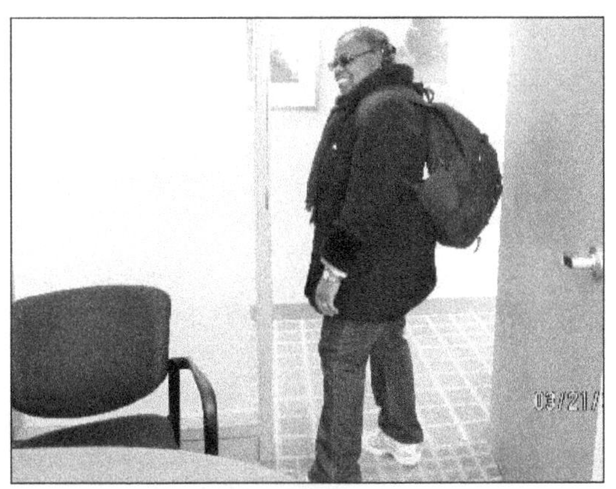

STUDENT ME WITH BACKPACK LOADED WITH BOOKS

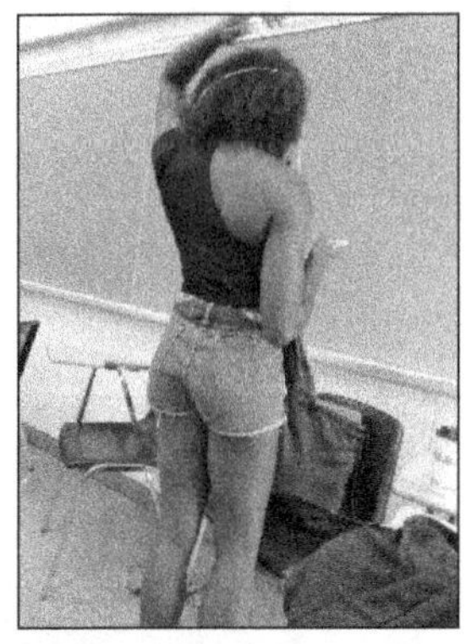

SUMMER WEAR ON CAMPUS

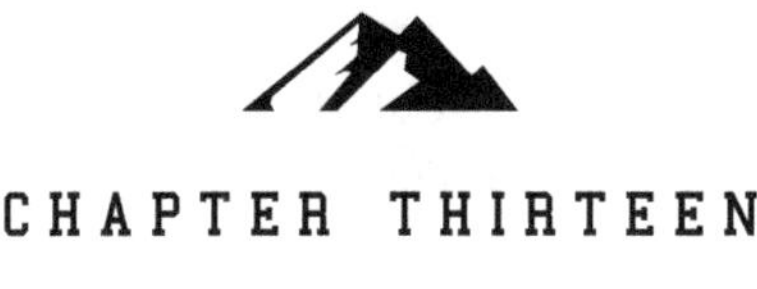

CHAPTER THIRTEEN

Group Work

"Work hard, be kind and amazing things will happen."
—CONAN O'BRIEN

One important criterion for me to attend York U. was to be among people. I craved the interaction between students, professors, and teaching assistants. Attending university made me feel alive from the moment I walked the seven minutes from home to the bus stop, to the moment I sat on the bus, to the moment I arrived on campus. The people and their movements added a dimension to life. As I searched the directories looking at courses to register for, I observed that some classes offered tutoring online. I had no interest in that format and refused to register for any of them.

In-person classes allowed me to see my classmates, hear them, observe them, and even form friendships with some of them; however, I soon discovered that millennials are difficult to befriend.

Group work became an important aspect of teaching in post-secondary education institutions. According to a study by the University of Waterloo, "Group work can be an effective method to motivate students, encourage active learning, and develop key critical-thinking, communication, and decision-making skills."

Professors seemed to love the idea of group work. They placed us in small groups in several of my classes, forcing us to work together. But after organizing the groups, they abdicated their responsibilities and never bothered to check to see how the students were doing. I soon learned that group work is a crapshoot. Of all the groups I had been a part of (I'd been a part of several), only one worked well, and I had championed it. One or two students in these groups always did very little work, or none at all. The issue that annoyed me most about group work was: whether students contributed or not they received the same grade as the other group members who did all the work.

Let me share a few of these stories:

During Digital Media in the Humanities, Professor Irons placed me in a group with Cory, a black eighteen-year-old boy from Grenada, and a nineteen-year-old boy from India, to work on a project. The body language of the Indian boy told me immediately that he did not wish to work with us. The professor provided the details of the project the groups should undertake. We were to write a script, then convert it into a video or a PowerPoint presentation. First, we had to prepare a storyboard that she would review and advise if we were on the right track. "Oh, brother! I can concoct a short story and write a script, no problem there. But make a storyboard? What the heck is that? Make a movie? I know nothing about these things," I thought. I'd watched many PowerPoint presentations in the corporate world but had never prepared one myself. I promptly volunteered to concoct a short story and write the script, hoping my two young partners would undertake the more technical jobs.

At the next class, Professor Irons announced that the Indian student had some personal issues to deal with, and he had withdrawn from the course. It meant the other groups had three members, while Cory and I had to do our project by ourselves. Not only that, I could have betted my pension cheque that I was the least technological person in the class. Whatever possessed me to take the digital media course?

Sitting on the bus heading home that evening, I wrote a short story and emailed it to Cory later that night. I employed the theme of "pursuing dreams." The story was about Dave Moody, a boy who grew up on a farm in rural Ontario, a real country bumpkin. He had gone on a field trip with his class to the big city, Toronto, for the first time to visit the Ontario Science Centre. He immediately fell in love with the gadgets and paraphernalia he had seen there. The planetarium especially fascinated him. After the trip, Dave became obsessed with science and pursued it relentlessly in high school and in university. He won several science project competitions. Dave graduated from university at the top of his class and became valedictorian that year. NASA eventually recruited him, and he trained to become an astronaut. Dave travelled to space. Afterwards, he toured Canada and the United States and delivered speeches to high school and college students, encouraging them to pursue their dreams as he had done.

Professor Irons offered to conduct a workshop on storyboarding via Skype. I had never used Skype and had no intention of doing so then. I suggested to Cory that we search the Internet for articles on how to prepare a storyboard. We should also search for free images we could use to bring our story to life—pictures of farm equipment, farmhouses, barns, science projects, award trophies, and graduation pictures. After all, wasn't everything on the Internet?

I found a helpful storyboard template on a website and used it to prepare a storyboard for the professor. Since I was not skilled in drawing, I added clip art to demonstrate some of the main points in the story. Cory was like a sponge; I had to squeeze him to get any response. He did not communicate with me or provide any of the items suggested. What was the lad thinking? Professor Irons had assigned 40 percent of our marks, the biggest component of the course, to this multimedia narrative project. Did Corey want to pass the course? Did he assume that I would do all the work? I knew my grade (no less than a B) depended on us putting together a first-class presentation. But it seemed that I couldn't rely on Cory.

Desperate and disillusioned, I contacted Donna, my favourite cousin, in Rochester, New York. She was a manager with an insurance company and did presentations regularly. I asked her to walk me through how to prepare a PowerPoint presentation. We spoke on the phone while I sat before my computer, and she sat before hers. Donna patiently guided me through the process, screen by screen. She taught me to add sound, insert pictures, and make the slides appear on the screen like a wheel, plus use fly-in, float-in, fade out, and other methods.

Years earlier, when I'd written blog articles, I had discovered a website that allowed you to download hundreds of free pictures without infringing on copyrights. I visited the site and found some of the most appropriate, colourful farm images that would bring Dave Moody's story to life. I downloaded the pictures and prepared the PowerPoint, adding brief captions to each slide. I timed the movement of the slides so that the presentation would remain within the three minutes Professor Irons had allowed each group.

I suspected some of my tech-savvy classmates would make brilliant little movies, so I wanted at least one slide to appear like a movie to compete with them. I found a video of one of the launchings of the space shuttle Atlantis and had a friend capture ten seconds of the launch on film. I incorporated it into the PowerPoint as the introductory slide to my story. The launch added drama to the presentation. I wrote a brief script to represent a part of the speech Astronaut Dave would have given to students as he travelled on his speaking tours. I asked one of my church brothers to read it, standing at the podium after one Sunday service. I filmed him reading and incorporated the film into the presentation. I reviewed and edited the PowerPoint, reducing it to three minutes, then forwarded a copy to *lazy* Cory. He came alive then. He was impressed. I assigned him to write a short script to narrate to the class during our presentation. He did, and that was his total contribution to the project.

On the day of the presentations, I expected some groups in the class to present movies, and they did. Some were quite good. Professor Irons and my classmates were impressed by the PowerPoint Cory and I presented. It had a moral, it had heart, it had passion, and the imagery was superb. The professor gave us an A, which boosted our marks for the entire course.

Months after the course ended, I was surprised to bump into Cory twice on campus. The university had a large student population, over fifty thousand, so there was a good chance that you would never see a classmate again from one of your courses unless you pursued the same major. Cory greeted me with warm hugs as if I were his long-lost aunt.

The course Understanding Food consisted of lectures and in-class group work. Since about five hundred students attended lectures, the professor placed us in several groups and assigned them letters. My group of five was assigned AQ. At the first group-work meeting, only the male student among us and I attended. At the next two meetings two students and I attended. The fourth week, a female Indian student, mouth filled with metal, came for the first time. We had to do a group assignment that week—we had one every second week. The Indian student had a tablet. We asked her to search for information about one assignment question while another student looked up information on the second question. The Indian student did nothing. She could not find anything using her tablet. She never attended another group-work class. I inquired if she had dropped the course. One student who had spoken to her by telephone explained that she had not dropped the course. She had not attended classes because her father could not drive her to the campus! The male student missed a few classes, and explained that he had to work. At the end of the course, my group received 80 percent for the in-class assignments. All five members received that same grade, even the Indian student who attended one group-work class only, and contributed nothing.

In early September 2019, I entered one of the Curtis Lecture halls on the second floor. Seats were arranged theatre-style, and I sat in the first seat in the third row. I was early as usual, so I observed the students as they entered. They were all millennials except one woman, about fifty-five. I later befriended her. By start time, about one hundred students filled the room. The class was Urbanization and Community Action, a course that explores the history of urbanization in Canada and how it helped shape inequity and social exclusion in society. It was my first social science course, and it encompassed two semesters. The classes had two parts, a lecture and a tutorial. Somehow, the professor arranged it ass-backwards because, after the introductory class, I had tutorials first, then the lectures.

Professor Jane was a petite, shapely woman, bleach-blond, about fifty. She breezed into the room five minutes late. She wore tight jeans and a tight sweater that emphasized her voluptuous breasts. Her favourite word was the f-word, which punctuated many of her sentences. She had a terrible hacking cough, probably from smoking. She claimed that her heritage was part Scottish and part aboriginal. During one lecture, when she delved into the history of Canada and the treatment meted out to the aboriginals by the Europeans, she burst into tears. The class held its breath and waited for her to recover.

We had a lot to cover during that six-credit course, and Professor Jane expected us to read twenty-five to thirty pages of text for each class. Despite the time constraint of the lectures, she spent a good chunk of her time talking about herself and her ex-boyfriends. She seemed desperate to identify with the young students. In one class, she told us about her new dog. She showed us a picture of the lovable pooch on her cell phone, then exclaimed, "You people know more about my life than the people I date!" Although she frequently digressed during lectures, we read a lot about the subject and completed assignments, indicating that we kept up with the course. She divided the class into small groups in tutorials, and during those times, we spent the time telling her what we thought instead of her teaching us.

Urbanization and Community Action proved to be a fascinating course. We began by examining early humans, who were hunters, gatherers, and nomadic. We moved through how cities progressed and developed, Jericho being the oldest-known city at about ten thousand years old. We marched through historical times and discussed the impact of the industrial revolution on cities. We discussed the major modern cities like New York, London, Beijing, and Paris.

At the beginning of the second semester, Professor Jane instructed us to form groups of three or four. The millennials quickly created groups with other millennials. I was never a first-choice pick in any group formation. I had gotten to know Michelle, the fifty-five-year-old woman, and she came to join me. Claudia, a pretty Italian girl with black curls cascading over her head, found she was alone and walked from the far end of the room to join us. We were the leftovers of the class. Professor Jane gave us the assignment to prepare a class presentation based on a summary of the readings we had done from the beginning of the course up to the time we presented. We were to connect what we had read to other society issues and provide her with a written copy of our presentations.

Each group had to select the date they would present. Never wanting to be first or last, I quickly chose February 13th, a date in the middle of the schedule. I learned during the first semester of the course that Claudia was carrying a full course load, and she also worked part-time. Michelle also undertook a full course load, desperate to earn her degree and eventually obtain a decent job. Remembering my previous painful experiences with group work and knowing that my group mates had the burden of other courses, I felt I had to take charge. I immediately volunteered to summarize all the readings we had covered and highlight the main topics. It allowed us to connect the topics to issues in society. We agreed to focus our presentation on the social matter of homelessness in the Greater Toronto Area. I assigned Claudia to research the multifaceted causes of homelessness and Michelle to research which governments—federal, provincial, and municipal—were doing something to alleviate homelessness. I would research three primary nongovernmental organizations (NGOs) that supported the homeless.

Michelle and Claudia appreciated my offer. During the semester, we communicated regularly by email to make sure each group member kept on schedule with their part of the work. I applied my previously learned PowerPoint skills and made a brief introductory presentation with images depicting: the early man as hunter and gatherer, aboriginal peoples who had inhabited Canada for centuries, the arrival of white men as traders, rural agricultural Canada, and the first two major cities, Montreal and Toronto.

On our presentation day, I showed the PowerPoint pictorial introduction; then Michelle, Claudia, and I delivered our verbal presentations. They were professional, informative, and linked effectively with the social issue of homelessness in the Greater Toronto Area. Professor Jane applauded us. We earned an A.

* * *

It was a bitterly cold day, the last class for February. The wind blew snow across my path as I crossed Steeles Avenue from the bus stop and headed for the campus grounds. A new Toronto Transit subway station built on campus, opened officially in the fall of 2018. After it opened, the York Region Transit buses, my means of commute that had driven onto the university campus for years, were no longer permitted on the grounds, hence my trek from Steeles Avenue.

The wind was so strong that it blew the heavy hood of my winter coat off my head and onto my shoulders. It made no sense to put it back up just to have it blown off again. Luckily, I wore a togue under the hood; it kept my head warm. I trudged across a field as I'd done all semester, only now the grass was covered in more than two feet of snow. Slowly, I placed one foot in front of the other, sinking deeper into the snow as I struggled to move forward. Words of the Christmas carol, "Good King Wenceslas," flashed into my mind:

Mark my footsteps, good my page.
Tread thou in them boldly
Thou shalt find the winter's rage
Freeze they blood less coldly.

Unfortunately, there were no footsteps in the virgin snow for me to follow. I created my own hard-to-plod path. When I crossed the field to enter the Founders College building, I was experiencing excruciating pain in my hips and knee. My arthritis was raging. I had to stop.

To add insult to injury, the back door of the Founders College building, where I usually entered, was locked. I plodded across a small courtyard and entered the building on the lower level through a door that took me into the domain of the janitorial staff. No one was in sight. I sat on the second step at the bottom of a stairway, panting and huffing. From one of the three small compartments at the front of my backpack, I removed a pouch that performed the jobs of a makeup bag and pencil case. I retrieved a small plastic bottle of Tylenol Extra Strength and swallowed two pills. I washed them down by gulping two mouthfuls of water from the York U. water bottle I always carried in my backpack. I prayed to God to ease my pain and help me make it to my classroom.

Tears welled up in my eyes and rolled down my cheeks. Why was I doing this? Why was I suffering to attend a class? The small voice inside my head whispered: "Be strong. Remember texture, remember staving off dementia, remember inspiring your grandsons, remember you crave knowledge." After five minutes (it felt like thirty), the pain began to subside. I painstakingly climbed the fifteen steps that led to the first floor and exited the building. I crossed a small field and entered York Lanes.

I was sitting just outside the classroom on the third floor of the Accolade West building, talking to Claudia and waiting for our class to start, when Michelle arrived. At 3:15 p.m., Claudia heard a ding and checked her cell phone. Professor Jane had just sent an email advising the students that she had cancelled the tutorial and lecture for that day. She did not provide any explanation.

Understandably, I was pissed off. I had struggled to plod through two feet high snow and suffered excruciating pain to arrive for class, and early at that. Professor Jane had waited until fifteen minutes before our class should begin to inform us she was not coming. Who does that?

CHAPTER FOURTEEN

Then There Was Ross

"Be slow to fall into friendship; but when thou art in, continue firm and constant."

—SOCRATES

Halfway through the degree program, I signed up for the English course Prose Narrative. The Academic Calendar for the Faculty of Liberal Arts & Professional Studies specified that all students majoring in English must take a class that included pre-eighteenth-century literature. This course included literature from the 1600s. The brief outline on the website stated that it is "An introduction to the formal techniques and generic patterns that have governed prose narrative in English since the 16th century to the present time." A more detailed description mentioned that the course focuses on unifying possibilities of narrative and its main principles—plot, characterization, reader engagement, and thematic emphasis.

On the first day of the class, I arrived half an hour early. The classroom on the third floor of the Stong College building, arranged to hold about fifty students, was empty. I plopped my derriere on a seat at the end of the third row. Shortly after, a woman in a wheelchair motored into the room. I observed that the university administrators did their best to accommodate disabled persons. They had constructed ramps on buildings all over the campus, installed low elevator buttons, and placed big metal buttons the size of saucers on many doors so that disabled persons could open them by pressing the buttons with their hands or even elbows. I assumed the woman in the wheelchair was a student and asked if I could help.

"No, thank you," she said. "I'll just set up my PowerPoint. I'm Rachelle."

Rachelle was the name on the course description. My eyes popped open.

She was the professor for my course!

Professor Rachelle looked like a teenager. She was slim, wore black-rimmed glasses, and had her hair in a ponytail. Her wheelchair was the Cadillac of wheelchairs. It was motorized and adjustable to different heights, with hand rests and a headrest. Her feet were turned inward. It appeared that she couldn't walk.

I experienced the typical prejudice that able-bodied people initially feel when they come in contact with a disabled person. Weird questions popped into my head. Would I understand her when she lectured? Would she be able to control the class? Would she mark our papers on time? She was assigned to teach the entire class in a room on the third floor of the Stong building and to conduct a tutorial for half of the class in another building. How difficult would it be for her to move from one classroom to the next?

Within ten minutes, Professor Rachelle had her PowerPoint presentation up and ready to roll. The first slide on the white screen welcomed the students to the course. Shortly before the lecture started, a pudgy man about my age, wearing tortoiseshell glasses, walked in. He scanned the room, then came and sat beside me. We exchanged hellos. His name was Ross. He had blue-grey eyes and hair grey throughout, long, curling at the nape of his neck. Five minutes into the lecture, a woman of about sixty-five with grey hair, wearing large-framed glasses that were popular in the 1980s, burst into the room like the gust of a hurricane. She dragged a suitcase on wheels behind her and promptly pushed her way to the middle of the front row, disturbing the students at one end. Professor Rachelle ignored her and continued the lecture.

Prose Narrative was the first class I attended with three seniors. In fact, I had been the only senior citizen in all of my classes until then. Some classes had a few middle-aged students dressed in business suits who attended during working hours but never seniors. The woman with the suitcase interrupted Professor Rachelle several times, asking her to repeat what she'd just said. She asked ridiculous questions that had nothing to do with the lecture. Ross and I exchanged glances and even laughed a few times.

"It's people like her who make seniors look bad," Ross whispered.

"You are so right," I whispered back.

The millennials looked up to the ceiling. I knew they wondered if the woman had all her faculties.

At the end of the lecture, Ross and I took the elevator together to ground level, then strolled to Vari Hall. The hall is a conical structure that interconnects with three buildings. Inside the rotunda, you look up two storeys. The walls are panelled with maple wood and strips of brown mahogany wood. The common space has built-in benches all around and an attractive information counter in the middle. Several display cases made from glass stood at the right, showcasing awards that celebrate faculty members' achievements. We sat quietly on a bench and ate our lunches. Our tutorial, scheduled to begin an hour after the lecture, would be held in one of the Vari Hall classrooms. Our teaching assistant would be Oliver.

Ross and I hung out together as the semester continued. Sometimes we sat at a table in the food court and other times on a bench in Vari Hall. Every topic was grist for our conversation mill. We shared information about our lives, former occupations, children, charity work, and passions. I learned that he was a retired teacher. He had a BA in history but decided to pursue an English degree this time. He was divorced, and his ex-wife had been an alcoholic. After the divorce, he lived the life of a single parent, taking care of his two children. I grew to like Ross, his easygoing manner, and his honesty. We became good friends. He drove an old lady weekly to do her shopping, the sign of a charitable man. I admired that about him.

Oliver, our teaching assistant, was a PhD candidate. While he guided our tutorials well, he was not an English major. He tended to ramble on about academic subjects too highfalutin for first-year students, the majority of the class. Ross usually sat beside me in tutorials. Whenever Oliver rambled, he would grab my notebook and scribble, “What was that all about?” We would exchange smiles and then focus back on Oliver. I felt like we were two naughty children in elementary school.

When the time came for us to write our first essay, Oliver provided three topics. We had to select one. He generously offered to review our thesis statements before we wrote our essays. That night, I stayed up late selecting the topic to write on, crafting a couple of thesis statements and editing them until I was satisfied with one. We had two weeks to submit our essays. I developed great confidence in writing essays after Professor Winter entered my essay into a competition. But every essay is different, and every professor or teaching assistant focuses on a different aspect. I wanted Oliver to indicate that I was on the right track and wasted no time. I emailed him my draft thesis statement the next day. Two days later, Oliver returned it with comments on how I could improve it and suggested how to defend the ideas. When I submitted my polished essay two weeks later, I felt confident I had done a great job. I received an A for my efforts.

* * *

Ross and I sat in our regular spot on a bench in Vari Hall after Professor Rachelle’s lecture. We were waiting to attend our tutorial. He complained that he was angry with Oliver.

“Why are you angry with the TA? What did he do?” I asked.

"He gave me a low mark for my essay. I have an appointment to see him after tutorial today to talk about the grade he gave me. He has to change it."

Hearing the venom in Ross's voice, I recalled the incidents Michelle, the teaching assistant of my first course, had experienced when students threatened her. Ross was behaving like those students, exhibiting the entitlement syndrome—I deserve better. Why did he not think about his grade as I had about mine? Oliver gave him a low mark based on his assessment of the essay. Why not ask Oliver to show him ways to improve his approach for future papers instead of demanding a better grade? Ross did not attend the next lecture or tutorial. He telephoned me a week later to say that Oliver refused to change the grade on his essay, that he hated him, and that he had withdrawn from the course. I had not figured Ross to be a quitter. Why drop the class because of a low mark on an essay? I suspected something else might be going on with Ross. He had taught school; he ought to know that a low grade signified the work was not good enough.

It was unfortunate that Ross withdrew from the course. Prose Narrative proved to be fabulous. We explored texts that included *The Man in the Moone*, published in 1638 and known as the first science fiction novel, Jane Austen's *Northanger Abbey*, Charlotte Bronte's *Jane Eyre*, Virginia Woolf's *To the Lighthouse,* Michael Ondaatje's *Running in the Family*, and more.

Professor Rachelle was an organized, punctual, and well-prepared teacher who shared knowledge freely. She dashed from lectures to tutorials in her wheelchair like a fire truck on a call. I tried to follow her one day to the elevator after a class. She left me in her dust! Without using words Professor Rachelle taught me a valuable lesson: do not prejudge people by their appearance and mobility status. Being handicapped does not mean they are brain-dead. Of all the professors I had at York U., she was one of the best. I articulated this in the survey that students completed after each course.

* * *

York U. offered a lot of leeway for students to withdraw from courses. Professors usually included information about the last day to drop a class without receiving a grade in their syllabus documents. It alarmed me that one of the courses I took, lasting from January 4th to April 8th, allowed students to withdraw up to March 12th. That meant a student could have attended a class for two months before dropping the course. They were responsible for officially withdrawing from the course via the registration system. The university would place a W on their transcripts, but it would not affect their grades. If students stopped attending classes and did not de-register, an F would appear on their transcript and affect their grade point average. Withdrawing from a course after attending classes for two months seemed like a colossal waste of time and effort. The information provided insight into why some students took longer than the allotted time to earn their degree and why some had excessive debts.

I never dropped a course during my entire studies. The thought of trying out a course by attending a few classes to see if I liked it or the professor never crossed my mind. Some students attended certain classes because they liked a professor, had heard good things from their peers about a professor, or read positive reviews online about a professor.

My modus operandi was: I read the course description carefully, made sure it interested me, and I wanted to learn more about the subject; then I registered. It mattered not whether the professor was a turd or a nice guy. Truth be known, I've never inquired about or checked out any professor online before registering for a course. The moment I clicked the "add course" link, I was committed to that course. There was no turning back for me at that point.

I recalled a story that demonstrated the extent to which some students will go to decide on courses to take. I continued to live a regular social life while attending York U. and went to the delightful wedding of the daughter of a couple in my church family. At the reception, held under a large white tent, guests were assigned to tables. I sat beside a gentleman my age whom I did not know. We introduced ourselves and struck up a conversation. His name was

Larry. I learned that he was an economics professor at a major university. Since I was a senior citizen student, we swapped stories about our experiences as teacher and student at university. Larry shared some hard-to-believe stories. One was about a male student who had attended one of his classes. He also attended classes in every faculty for an entire semester during one year. Naturally, the professors exchanged notes, and when Larry heard about this, he asked the student why he was doing it. The student replied that he was unsure about which degree to pursue and felt that attending classes in each faculty would help him to decide. In the end he opted to study engineering at a university in a remote area of another province.

The world and its systems can be so manipulative that sometimes it is impossible to tell the truth from fiction. For example, a few months after I'd completed Law and Morality in Literature and Culture, I received an email from the professor who taught that course. He asked me to go to a particular website and write a positive review about him. He explained that he was having a problem with a male student and his buddies. They had undertaken a poison-pen campaign against him and written several negative reviews about the professor as revenge because the student had received a low grade for his course. It shocked me to hear that a student could be vindictive enough to resort to such lengths to damage a professor's reputation merely because he had not received the mark he wanted. Are these the people entering the workforce? What will they do when they receive a less-than-stellar job review? The poor professor had to expend his time trying to counteract negative information instead of utilizing it to prepare his lectures. I wondered if the student ever felt joy from doing such a disgusting thing.

Long before the request, I had concluded that the professor was passionate about the subject he taught and even more passionate about *Kafka,* one of the texts we studied. He was also generous with his time. Three students and I had missed the first two lectures and could not obtain notes from our classmates. The professor offered to remain behind after the third lecture and brought us up-to-date on the topics he had covered. I appreciated him for his kindness and thoughtfulness. I knew he also valued me because as I handed him my final exam booklet, he said, "Good luck with all your endeavours, Yvonne. It was a pleasure having you in my class."

I thought it ironic that a professor who taught a course about law and morality, and showed us how Martin Luther was ostracized because he pointed out that selling indulgences by the Catholic Church was immoral, was being persecuted by a student. It seemed that the student had not learned anything about morals. I wrote a positive, truthful review about the professor and posted it on the website.

I was pleased that Ross was not mean-spirited and never threatened the teaching assistant. We never attended another course together because the English courses he took were ones I had already done; however, we kept in touch and still communicate today.

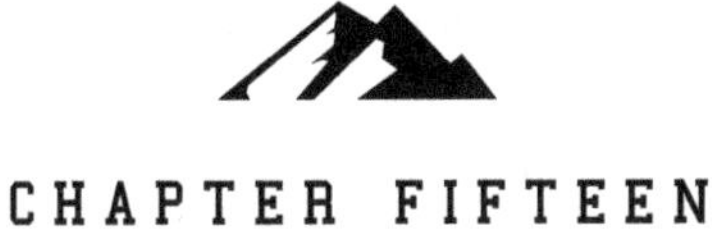

CHAPTER FIFTEEN

Covid-19 Drove Classes Online

"Technology is not a silver bullet. It's only as good as the teachers ... using it as one more tool to help inspire, and teach, and work through problems."

—BARACK OBAMA

It seemed that the stars were once more not aligned in my favour to achieve my goal of earning an English degree, for not long after the dreary protracted strike on campus ended, the World Health Organization (WHO) declared the novel coronavirus (COVID-19) outbreak a global pandemic on March 11, 2020.

At that time, I was engrossed in Urbanization and Community Action, with only three lectures, three tutorials, a group assignment, and the final exam remaining. The day following the declaration by WHO, Professor Jane sent the students an email stating, "As requested by the Dean's office, we will be switching to an online format for this course." She instructed us where to go on the university's website and how to submit our group assignment. COVID-19 was finally impacting the university, and the administration made changes quickly.

I had borrowed *Edge of Empire: Postcolonialism and the City* by Jane M. Jacobs from the Scott Library to gather information for my small group's presentation. Now students could no longer enter the campus. How could I return the book? I definitely did not want to incur any fines because the university prohibited me from doing so. The library's personnel became aware and immediately extended the return date to several months out. Later, when the time expired and COVID-19 continued to rage, they renewed it again.

Since I had never wanted to do online courses, I was relieved that only three lectures and tutorials would be taught by that method. I signed into my student account online and checked the progress of my degree. Eighteen more credits were required to cross the finish line. I suddenly realized that my goal for 2020 was unachievable. There would be no seventieth birthday present and no celebration party. Oh, well, they say when life throws you lemons, you should make lemonade. I had not engraved my graduation date in concrete; it was adjustable. Besides, it was evident that you don't always get what you want when you want it. And yes, it would have been wonderful to give myself a seventieth birthday gift of an English degree. I reset my graduation date for 2021.

On the day and time of my first online class and one of the final three lectures in Urbanization and Community Action, instead of slipping on my backpack, dashing out the door, and walking seven minutes to catch the York Region Transit bus, I climbed the stairs to the second floor, entered my home office, and booted up my desktop computer. As I sat at the desk waiting for the computer to load up its programs, it suddenly hit me like a punch in the gut that for the remainder of the course, I would no longer bundle up and experience the brisk seven-minute walk between my home and the bus stop and the long walk between the classroom and the bus stop at Steeles Avenue. I would no longer see the commuters on the bus or listen in on their conversations. I would no longer sit in the lecture hall listening to Professor Jane speak and inject some of her personal escapades. I would no longer see my small group members, Claudia and Michelle—the only two people from the class I had bonded with—and I would no longer see any of my other classmates. It felt like someone had swiftly turned off a gushing fountain or like a glowing candle had rudely been snuffed out.

I hadn't stepped on the scale for some time, too scared of what it might register, but I felt confident that I had lost five pounds, thanks to my commute and walking in the snow to and from Steeles Avenue to campus. Now that activity was over. What incentive would I need to walk?

The computer came alive with the programs loaded. I clicked on the York U. icon and entered my dashboard for the course. The class was supposed to be via Zoom. I clicked on the Zoom link. Nothing happened. After several tries, a message appeared on the screen: "the Zoom site is unavailable." The system had become overloaded. For the remainder of the course, Zoom remained unavailable. Professor Jane posted PDF copies of her lectures on the university's website. I read them several times and took notes. If students had questions, they had to send emails to the professor and wait a couple of days for answers.

Reading the lectures at home alone, tucked away in my office, I felt disconnected, like being on a deserted island separated from humanity, wading through unchartered waters. It was certainly no way to conduct a university course. The final exam, scheduled for April 2nd, would be open book. Open book! There they went again with these twenty-first-century ideas. How would a professor know that you had read the text and lectures and learned anything if you could read it while writing the exam? I soon understood that it was not as simple as I thought. Once you entered the portal for the exam, you had ninety minutes to answer all the questions. You could not sign out and reenter. In other words, if you had not read the text and lectures, you would never have had enough time to search for the answers. You had to have done the work to meet the timeline. Gosh! Contemporary ideas do work—sometimes.

Our final group assignment was due on April 9th. Since I had taken charge of the project, I combined the information I researched with materials from Michelle and Claudia into one document. I edited it, checking for spelling and grammatical errors and double-checking that the paragraphs flowed methodically. Satisfied with the finished product, I submitted the document online.

I sent my teammates the following email:

> *Okay, my classmates! I submitted our assignment at 1:37 p.m.—Yippee!*
> *I am attaching what was finally submitted. I made a few grammatical changes. I also formatted the references in alphabetical order as Michelle suggested, and I gave the prof her title—Dr. We all worked hard on this, so I expect an "A." We will see. Good luck to you both, and all the best with your studies.*
> *Yvonne*

Michelle responded by email minutes later:

> *Oh, my goodness, you both are awesome...it's done*👌👌👌
> *Yes, have a wonderful summer!*

Claudia responded later by email:

> *Thank you, Yvonne!*
> *Best of luck to you ladies; enjoy your summer*😄

Professor Jane did not provide students with their test results until sometime in June. By then, we were engrossed in our summer courses. I prayed that COVID-19 would be vanquished soon, allowing students to return to in-person classes to complete their degrees. Little did I know that the pandemic would fume on and on, attaining peaks and valleys for a couple of years.

A year after I had completed Urbanization and Community Action, the library book remained on my dining table. I wanted it out of the house. I contacted the library by phone to inquire if I could drop it off. The answer was no! They extended the due date several times, and it remained in my possession for nineteen months.

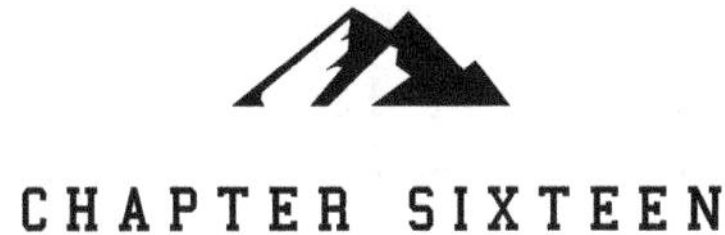

CHAPTER SIXTEEN

Literature and Drugs

"Addiction begins with the hope that something 'out there' can instantly fill up the emptiness inside."
—JEAN KILBOURNE

Call me naïve if you like, but I must admit that until about twenty years ago, I knew very little about drug addicts. Raised by grandparents in Manchester, a rural part of Jamaica, I never heard about anyone or saw anyone who was a drug addict. The villagers were clean-living people who believed in God, and the church played a fundamental role in the community. Alcohol—rum—was an important, celebratory drink served at events like weddings and funerals but drunk in moderation. A few rum heads lived in the district; they bothered no one, and everyone knew who they were.

After living in Canada and associating with many white Canadians, I learned that some have preconceived ideas that all Jamaicans know and smoke marijuana (ganja). They may have gotten this idea because people who sold it tended to haunt the resorts where these Canadians stayed when they visited the island.

I saw a marijuana plant for the first time in Toronto in 1977. My then-husband had made friends with a Trinidadian couple, and one Saturday evening, they invited us for dinner at their apartment. While Bev rustled up a meal in the kitchen, Len and my husband sat by the stereo and sorted records to play. I walked around the living room, admiring the houseplants. One particular plant attracted me because of its succulent, delicate green leaves. I turned to Len and asked him the name of it, thinking I would buy one for my apartment. He plucked his cigarette from his mouth, placed it on an ashtray near the stereo, and burst out laughing. The man laughed so hard I thought he would pee his pants.

Confused, I asked, "What's so amusing about my simple question?"

Bev rushed from the kitchen and stood beside him. They glowered at me as if I had arrived from Mars.

After Len regained his composure, he asked, "You really don't know what that plant is?"

"If I knew, I wouldn't have asked you, Len," I said.

"Shh, don't tell anyone," Len said. "It's marijuana."

Marijuana was illegal in Canada at that time. He could have knocked me over with one of the succulent green leaves of the plant. I laughed at my ignorance and confessed that I had never seen the plant before.

My only experience with marijuana had been fleeting, and I never actually saw it. The incident occurred while attending the College of Arts, Science, and Technology in Kingston. At the end of my last class on a Friday, six students piled into one car and headed for a beach on St. Thomas Road, just outside the city. We had sprawled out on blankets, relaxing, listening to the lapping of the waves, soaking up the last rays of sunshine, and enjoying music from a small stereo, when one of my classmates lit a spliff. We passed it around, each one taking puffs. But with six people smoking one spliff, I took only two draws. Bells did not peal, the hallelujah chorus did not play, and I felt nothing. That incident accounted for my entire experience with drugs.

* * *

In April 2020, five weeks after York U. locked down the campus because of the COVID-19 pandemic, I tried to register for a summer course. The university had switched all classes to online earlier, and they remained in that mode. I entered the code for the subject I wanted to take several times, but the online registration system knocked me out and gave messages that the class was restricted. I tried to register for another course and received a similar message. I became very concerned. There I was, trundling toward my seventieth birthday, still climbing the mountain, seeing the summit getting closer and closer as I hurtled toward achieving my goal of earning an English degree, only to come upon another hurdle. I had to earn six more credits from an English course to fulfill the requirements of my major. It did not matter if the class was a 2000-level or a 6000-level; I did not want the summer to end without earning six credits in English. An adage states that "Desperate times call for desperate measures." Well, desperation ran through my veins. I telephoned the English Department. Of course, no one was on-site to take my call, so I left a frantic message.

Kimberly replied: April 22 @yorku.ca

> *Good day Yvonne. I retrieved your voicemail (we all work from home). Please email me with the courses you would like to enroll in. Plus, with your excellent grades, have you thought of changing your Ordinary BA to an Honours BA? Congrats on your hard work. Please note that our 4th-year courses are for Honours BA students only as Ord. BA students do not require 4th-year courses.*
> *Cheers and stay safe, Kimberly*

I responded the same day with this email:

From: Blackwood
To: <@yorku.ca>

Subject: Re: English department voice mail message

Hello Kimberly, thanks for your response and kind words. I am retired; therefore, I do not want to do an Honours BA. The issue is: I only require 18 credits to complete the degree. I wanted to do at least a 6-credit course this summer. I need six more credits from an English course to comply with the requirements of my major. I know I do not have to do a 4000-level course; however, all the 3000-level English courses I'm interested in, were cancelled. I tried registering for AP/EN 4000.6 (My first choice) and AP/EN 4181.6, but both gave me messages stating seats are restricted and to call the office, hence my call. Is there any way you can get me registered for one of these courses? After being unable to do any summer courses last year because of the strike, I would hate to spend my summer doing only a 3-credit course.

Thanks for your help in advance.
Regards, Yvonne Blackwood

Kimberly responded with this email:

April 23 @yorku.ca:
Yvonne, I have given you permission for EN 4181 Section B. EN 4000 is full. Please enroll as soon as possible. Best of luck.
Cheers, and stay safe, Kimberly.

I tried to register for the course one more time and succeeded. I sent Kimberly another email to thank her.

* * *

The summer course that caused that rigmarole was Studies in Contemporary Literature: Writers and Drugs. It became my first course done entirely online. The course description promised that we would explore the connection between drugs and writing in various cultures, modern and premodern. My minute knowledge about the subject significantly heightened my interest in the course. Several questions swirled around in my head. Did writers take drugs in the past and in modern times? Did writers truly improve their writing by taking drugs? Who were the drug-taking authors? How did taking opioids help their writing? Naïve as I was, I knew enough that taking drugs was popular in the music world. Famous artists like Brian Wilson, David Bowie, Amy Winehouse, Natalie Cole, and Michael Jackson were said to be drug addicts; however, I did not know anything about drug-addicted authors.

The professor recommended four novels for the course—two written by Americans and two by Asians. The authors were all drug addicts. Interestingly, they used avatars as their protagonists; however, evidence showed that most of the information in the novels imitated their lives. We also read excerpts from two other books and several academic papers about drugs and their use in different cultures. The course would open my eyes to a new world and offer me a new high. I was keen to climb the mountain.

Monday, the first day of the course, was a disaster. Professor Bernstein sent the students an email apologizing that the website for the class was not yet active. She assured us that the university was doing everything possible to get it up and running. She attached narrated PowerPoint slides explaining the syllabus and the first two assignments. Our first journal entry was due on Wednesday. She advised us not to panic; it should be introductory writing to let her know a bit about us, and we could submit it on Thursday instead.

We began the course by examining *The Bacchae,* a play written by Euripides in 405 BCE. As the story goes, the people of Thebes had not recognized or adored Dionysus, son of the human mother Semele, and Zeus, the primary Olympian god, as a real god. Dionysus returned to Thebes to take revenge for the snub on King Pentheus, Agave, the king's mother, and Cadmus, the father of Agave—all members of Dionysus's family. He influenced the women of Thebes to establish a cult of Dionysus worshippers. Some women in the cult abandoned their children and roamed wild in the hills, carrying out bloody rituals after they became intoxicated with wine. The madness escalated, and Agave returned to the palace after a crazy night of wine drinking in the forest with the severed head of Pentheus, her son. She believed it was the head of a beast she had captured and expected Cadmus to applaud her and throw a party. He abhorred the deed.

Next, we examined an excerpt from Thomas De Quincey's *Confessions of an English Opium-Eater.* De Quincey penned sordid details about his life in the early 1800s, from the first time he took opium in 1804 while in college to becoming addicted to it. We also examined an excerpt from Aldous Huxley's *The Doors of Perception*, published in 1954. Huxley details how he took mescaline, a psychedelic drug processed from the peyote cactus used in indigenous religious ceremonies in North America for thousands of years. He took the drugs under the supervision of Humphry Osmond, a British psychiatrist, who documented everything Huxley felt, saw, and perceived while under the influence of the mescaline.

We probed Joan Didion's article, "Slouching Towards Bethlehem." In 1967, Didion journeyed to San Francisco and lived among hippies to learn firsthand about their lives and drug-taking habits. She did not take drugs; she made that clear in the article. Didion had much to say about hippies. Two things stood out blatantly: the variety of drugs the hippies took (she mentioned at least ten) and the ease of obtaining them, and how much hippies lacked language. It seemed that drugs had robbed them of the ability to express themselves.

They were unable to string words or sentences together. “Groovy” and “Peace and love” seemed all they could say.

* * *

By the time I had registered for Studies in Contemporary Literature: Writers and Drugs, I’d long since learned that outlines posted on the university’s website gave little detail about the courses. The syllabus document issued by the professor for this course provided a weekly description of what she planned for classes, including when we should read the books or articles and when assignments were due. A section titled “Assignment Guidelines” specified that students should prepare two podcast episodes; one due on May 25th, the other on July 30th.

A podcast! What the heck did a podcast have to do with a literature course? After that outburst (in my head), I calmed down and thought about it. I was attending York U. to learn and to find a way (*Tentanda via*), and I craved knowledge. If producing a podcast had to be done, then I should just do it. I read the instructions carefully. Students had to submit two podcast episodes based on the theoretical materials we read for the course, and each should include a discussion about one other kind of media.

I pounced on YouTube the week before the first podcast episode became due and spent hours researching how to produce a podcast. I found Anchor, a simple podcast app. The instructions were easy to follow, and you could edit errors after the recording. Anchor even included an extensive music catalogue, from classical to jazz, that you could add to the podcast.

I chose the theoretical piece, *The Doors of Perception* by Aldous Huxley, and wrote a script for the first podcast, modelling it as an interview between Huxley and a reporter. I searched the Internet, found a free picture of a mysterious door partially covered with ivy, and downloaded it. I practised recording the interview and realized that although my voice was okay as the interviewer, it was not suitable for Aldous Huxley. A male voice would be more appropriate. I contacted Rob, my son, and asked him to read the part of Huxley. He did a lousy job and knew it. He solicited Triscott, his father-in-law, who promptly agreed to read the part. He read it with a clear voice, and enunciated the words excellently. You would have thought he was an actor. Rob recorded the entire episode on his cell phone and forwarded it to me. I edited the recording, added the downloaded picture of the mysterious door as the cover for my podcast, and inserted snippets of mood music at the beginning and end. Satisfied with the result, I submitted the recording to Anchor. Shortly after, I received an email stating they had forwarded the podcast for distribution to Spotify and planned to submit it to Apple Podcasts and other listening platforms. My goodness! I could hardly believe it. Overnight, I became a podcaster! When the assignment came due, I submitted my script via a Word document to Professor Bernstein and included a link for the podcast. I felt confident the second episode would be easy to do, having gone through the process step by step.

Next, we read the novel *Junky* by William S. Burroughs, published in 1953. He published the story as a novel, but it included details from his own life. Lee, Burroughs's alter ego, narrated the story in the first person. He told the story of a life that was entirely absorbed in taking drugs, dealing drugs, and at times committing crimes to pay for his next fix. He exposed us to the underworld of drugs and its subculture, the camaraderie between users and dealers, the deprivation addicts endured, and the scams they contrived to obtain drugs when funds were lacking. Lee painted the most stirring, vivid images of addicts in their most vulnerable states—withdrawal, inability to cope, and near-death experiences. Doolie was one of his junkie cohorts, and Lee shared the information about his junk sickness:

> Doolie sick was an unnerving sight. The envelope of personality was gone, dissolved by his junk-hungry cells. Viscera and cells, galvanized into a loathsome insect-like activity, seemed on the point

> of breaking through the surface. His face was blurred, unrecognizable, at the same time, shrunken and tumescent.

We examined some of Allan Ginsberg's poetry. A known drug addict, Ginsberg wrote poetry that is raw, but gives a true sense of what it was like to be addicted to drugs. He began his poem "Howl" this way:

> I saw the best minds of my generation destroyed by madness, starving, hysterical, naked, dragging themselves through the negro streets at dawn looking for an angry fix, angelheaded hipsters burning for the ancient heavenly connection to the starry dynamo in the machinery of night…

In *Fear and Loathing*, published in 1971, Hunter S. Thompson used the avatar Raoul Duke to narrate the story. Duke, a magazine journalist, and his attorney, Doctor Gonzo, sped along the highway in a rented red Chevrolet convertible. They headed for Las Vegas, where Duke had the assignment to cover the 4th Annual Mint 400 Race, consisting of motorcycles and dune buggies. Before heading out, they stocked up on all kinds of drugs and booze—two bags of marijuana (grass), seventy-five pellets of mescaline, five sheets of high-powered blotter acid, cocaine, several uppers, downers, screamers, raw ether, and twenty-four amyls. They also bought a quart of tequila, a quart of rum, and a case of Budweiser. Duke described the trunk of the car as "A mobile police narcotics lab."

Duke and Gonzo arrived intoxicated at the Mint Hotel in downtown Las Vegas, where they had reservations, unable to communicate with the desk clerk to get checked in. Eventually, they obtained their room keys and spent the night boozing and taking drugs. The next morning, they could barely cope when they attended the start of the Mint 400 Race. Duke and his attorney left the race shortly after it started, so Duke had no coverage to write his assignment. They spent the rest of their time drinking and taking drugs. The pair got involved in several escapades and eventually left Las Vegas without completing any assignments. They remained high on drugs and were afraid that the police would arrest them the entire time.

* * *

In week three in June, I wrote and submitted two essays. I had developed confidence in essay writing but took nothing for granted. After all, Studies in Contemporary Literature: Writers and Drugs was a high-level course. I felt privileged to be accepted into it. I read all assigned texts carefully by applying the close reading skills acquired over five years. I dissected the essay questions to be sure I understood what the professor was asking for. I read and reread my essays, recorded myself reading them (a great way to detect errors), and edited them to near perfection—so I thought.

I received marks in the 70 percent range for each essay and was not thrilled, but did not demand any grade changes. I only wanted to do better. But I learned that in this harsh, cruel world, you must advocate for yourself. I did.

I sent the professor this email:

> **To:** b@yorku.ca
> **Subject:** Re: Improving Grades
>
> *Hello Professor,*
> *I have never argued with any of my professors about the grades I receive because I have always been satisfied with them. This email is not intended to argue about my marks, but as I complete one of my last three courses, I am becoming a bit frustrated that I have not been able to receive at least 80% for any of the assignments I have submitted so far. I read your comments on all my assignments*

carefully and tried not to repeat any errors etc., that you mentioned. I have also devoted the same amount of time and effort that I have done for all my courses. It appears, however, that I need to do more to achieve an "A," the goal I've aimed for. Could you provide some advice on what else I can do to improve my grade for the final assignments? I would much appreciate this.
Much regards,
Yvonne

The professor replied with this email:

b@yorku.ca
To: Blackwood

Hi Yvonne,
I'm sorry to know you've been disappointed with your grades, but I do understand; an A is always a worthy goal, though Bs are nothing to sneeze at! (They are still good or very good, and are at present the highest grades I have been awarding in this class). It can be hard, on reaching fourth-year courses, to find that work that previously received A's no longer necessarily do. The grading for fourth-year English courses is rigorous. A paper in this context will need an excellent thesis, a well-organized and well-supported argument, near-flawless language, and correct citations.
If you would send me your working thesis for your final paper, I will do my best to work with you to ensure that you have a solid foundation from which to work. You could also send me an outline for your essay: break your ideas down into their respective paragraphs including, in point form, the main

> *points you will make, and indicate what quotations from primary and secondary source material you will use. I will be happy to read this over and offer some feedback.*
> *Best wishes,*
> A. Bernstein

I appreciated the professor's response and took her up on her suggestion for my final essay at the end of July.

* * *

During the second half of the course, we immersed ourselves in the two novels *Candy* and *Taipei,* written by Asians. *Candy,* by Mian Mian, was published in 2003 and set in China. It tells the story of the agony of love, drugs, and becoming a writer. The novel begins with Hong, the protagonist, as a suicidal teenager. She left home and worked briefly as a nightclub singer, experiencing violence, alcoholism, and heroin addiction. She was committed to an institution for the criminally insane. Hong attempted suicide a few times. She had an obsessive, toxic love relationship with a man that lingered until the novel ended. Although Mian Mian published the story as a novel, Hong, the protagonist, echoed her lived experiences. Her character changed around the middle of the book when she started to write. Writing that began as therapy influenced how she saw the world and the concept of herself. It became a means by which Hong gained greater control over her emotions. It liberated her from addiction, and she became a writer.

As I studied these stories about writing and drugs, I asked these questions: Why did writers take opioids in the first place? No one knew in advance how drugs would affect them, so why take the chance? Most of the writers we studied seemed to have spiralled out of control at one point during their drug-taking journey, and while a few regained control, many never did.

The American Psychiatric Association provides an unequivocal definition of addiction on its website:

> Addiction is a complex condition, a brain disease that is manifested by compulsive substance use despite harmful consequence. People with addiction have an intense focus on using a certain substance such as alcohol or drugs, to the point that it takes over their life.

The four novels we studied proved that definition spot on.

At the end of the course, I returned to the questions I asked at the beginning: Did writers take drugs in the past and in modern times? Could writers truly improve their writing by taking drugs? How did taking drugs help their writing? Who were some of the other drug-taking authors besides the ones we studied?

The answers glared at me.

The texts for the course included both premodern and modern stories and showed clearly that some writers from both ages took drugs. In *The Bacchae*, dating back to 405 BCE, wine was the drug. Did drugs improve any author's writing? Research shows that some drugs, like cannabis, seemed to contribute to artistic production or at least enjoyment, while other drugs, like heroin, undermined it. I couldn't help thinking that some authors saw writing about drug addiction as a possible way to become famous or immortal (leaving their mark). After all, we are reading their stories today. De Quincey's drug addiction supplied him with a story he wrote and published that eventually gave him notoriety.

Despite my perception of why authors take drugs, these stories gave us food for thought. They provided exposure to a counterculture we might not have heard of, and insight into how taking different drugs affected their writing. Each author wrote that drugs had positive and negative elements, though mostly negative. The positive effect, however, is often related to creativity. Aldous Huxley boasted about the positive side and the beauty he experienced when he took mescaline. "I was seeing what Adam had seen the day of his creation—the miracle," he wrote. Paul Preciado reported that testosterone had a positive effect on his writing, that it gave him energy and focus. Hunter S. Thompson used mescaline, LSD, cocaine, alcohol, and other drugs and stated he saw hideous creatures and a blood-soaked carpet, and his attorney had vomiting bouts. In *Candy*, opioids helped the author to experience intensely. In each novel, taking drugs seemed to be a part of the rejection of, or rebellion against, social values and expectations.

Fascinated by the subject of addiction, I researched on my own to learn who are some of the other known drug-taking authors. I was shocked to discover the following:

Robert Louis Stevenson wrote sixty thousand words in six days while high on cocaine. Of course, we recall in *The Strange Case of Dr. Jekyll and Mr. Hyde*, the drug he mentioned was a white powdery substance.

Ken Kesey, it is said, was flying high on LSD when he wrote *One Flew Over the Cuckoo's Nest.*

Stephen King, a great horror story writer who churns out books like hotcakes, was addicted to cocaine.

Samuel Taylor Coleridge, best known for the poem "Kubla Kahn," was inspired to write it by an opium dream. The opium habit eventually caused his death.

Charles Dickens, the author of the novels *A Tale of Two Cities* and *Great Expectations,* was an opium addict.

CHAPTER SEVENTEEN

The Philosophers

"One cannot conceive anything so strange and so implausible that it has not already been said by one philosopher or another."
—RENÉ DESCARTES

I read Pearl Bailey's memoir, *Between You and Me,* when she published it in 1989. In it, Pearl tells the story that on the day she received an honorary degree from Georgetown University, without thinking, she spouted off during her thank-you speech that she might one day attend that institution. As they say, be careful what you wish for. A year later, Pearl entered Georgetown University as a freshman to pursue a BA in history. She graduated in 1985. At that time in Pearl's life, she had already gained fame and fortune. Why did she go back to school? She wrote, "I'm glad I 'went for it' and stuck with it to receive a college degree from Georgetown, at the age of sixty-seven!" Pearl also gave us her opinion on studying. "It's sacrifice and love intertwined. But most of all, it's a game of guts."

As I progressed through the English degree, Pearl's words reverberated in my head over and over, and I found myself doing some of the things she did. Her words were inspiring and oh-so-true. I sacrificed time, money, and simple pleasures to attend classes. I displayed guts when I stayed the course despite arthritic pain, terrible weather, and worse, an illness that later shook my world. My perseverance was seasoned with love, the love of learning. I craved knowledge.

Pearl's narration of her experience as a senior citizen student was infectious. When she wrote about the philosophers she had studied, you felt like you wanted to be in the classroom with her. I did not take any philosophy courses at York U. as a part of my studies. But as I emersed myself in Introduction to Literary Theory 1, I encountered some of the famous Greek philosophers Pearl had boasted about. The course description specified, "The course will introduce you to Homer's great epic, *The Iliad*, and the tradition of literary theory that tries to make sense of this achievement." We would examine how literary language does things and what they are by paying attention to literary figures like metaphors, similes, and the sublime. By the time I took this course, I had gained experience in close reading and knew numerous literary devices.

Homer had heard the tale about Troy and its war. He composed his epic poem, *The Iliad*, as a collection of stories combined into one unified story about 700 BCE. In a nutshell, the poem narrates this story: Helen, the wife of Menelaus, was abducted by Paris, one of the sons of King Priam of Troy, when he was a guest in the house of Atreus. Menelaus was the ruler of Sparta and the brother of King Agamemnon of Mycenae. Duty to family motivated Agamemnon to fight to get Helen back. He was also determined to vindicate the honour of the Greeks because it was paramount in the society at the time. Agamemnon felt that he and Menelaus would have no honour and appear weak if they did not seek revenge. They declared war on Troy, and a coalition of Greek allies, including Achilles, accompanied them in battle. But Zeus and the other Olympian gods interfered, and the war dragged on for ten years.

The text of *The Iliad* contained over six hundred pages, and it took three lectures to complete our review. Professor Valihora declared that *The Iliad* is a monument; it overwhelms you every time you read it. I read it for the first time, and considering that the text was composed in the seventh century, I couldn't help being awed by it. It certainly overwhelmed me. The words on the pages were electric. Homer crafted them to allow you to feel what he wanted you to feel. In the Homeric similes, some of them twelve lines long, he used pastoral images to compare situations in the battle, creating vivid and fascinating imagery.

I observed some interesting issues in the story: several beautiful women became the grandest prizes for the warriors to possess, and it didn't matter if they were married; gods had intimate relations with humans; parallels to events in the Bible, for example, the washing of hands and sacrificing animals to gods. Of course, the Hebrew Bible existed long before Homer recited his epic poem.

Next, we examined the first thirty chapters of the book of Genesis. The professor recommended we use the King James Version as it is known for its poetry. It was the third course I had taken in which the Bible played a key role. I began to appreciate it more, not just spiritually, but enjoying the crafting of the words on the pages, the literature. She stated that we could read the Bible in four ways: literal—the events literally happened; figurative/metaphorical—one thing stands for another; accommodation—how you write down the words and thoughts of God; typological—you read the text toward a goal. Professor Valihora drew some comparisons between *The Iliad* and the thirty chapters of Genesis that we read: In *The Iliad*, God represents nature. In Genesis, God created nature. It is subservient to the divine God. Homer crafted a story about an incident that occurred in the past. The author of Genesis recorded a story that happened thousands of years ago by employing several literary techniques to paint a vivid picture; Homer did similarly.

My experience learning about Greek philosophers was different from Pearl Bailey's. Her focus was on history; I pursued an English degree and focused on language. Introduction to Literary Theory 1 approached some of the great philosophers by exploring their understanding of language, words on a page, and opinions about *The Iliad.*

In Plato's *The Republic X,* he was concerned about emotions. He opined that when poets like Homer imitated a hero mourning and presented long speeches of lamentation or beat their breasts, listeners felt pleasure and became absorbed in the story. They then followed in sympathy and praised the poet. Plato believed that poetic imitation produced the effects of pleasure, desire, and pain of the mind, and those emotions should be controlled, thus allowing people to be better and happier. It seemed that he was not a fan of Homer. He also claimed that philosophy was better than any other discipline.

In *Poetics,* Aristotle discussed poetry. He asserted that poets are similar to painters or other visual artists; they created mimesis. He stated that many epic poets made plots like histories; Homer did this in *The Iliad.* Aristotle emphasized that a poet's job is not to say what did happen but the sort of thing that would happen, what is possible according to the law of probability or necessity.

But it was Longinus who educated me the most. In his treatise, "Longinus: On Sublimity," he wrote to Postumius Terentianus, a young colleague, to extoll the virtues of writing sublime literature. He elucidated the primary elements required to write sublime prose and poetry.

"Sublimity is a kind of eminence or excellence of discourse. It is the source of the distinction of the very greatest poets and prose writers and the means by which they have given eternal life to their own fame," Longinus wrote.

My goodness! Which writer wouldn't want to acquire such a skill? I became glued to the text after that opening statement, earnest to learn the sources of sublimity. Longinus enumerated the five primary requirements for his friend:

The power to conceive great thoughts
Strong and inspired emotion
Certain kinds of figures of speech (he listed those later)
Noble diction
Dignified and elevated word arrangement

I thought long and hard about these requirements and concluded that the first two ideas were not as simple as they sounded. What are great thoughts? Do we all conceive great thoughts? It seems we do not. Longinus further stated that people whose thoughts and habits are trivial and servile all their lives cannot produce great thoughts. Aha? I guess he hadn't read the Bible. Miracles do happen! What should one regard as strong and inspired emotion? There are so many emotions. How do we know which ones are strong and inspired? Longinus listed pity, grief, and fear as emotions that have a lower effect and are divorced from sublimity. He praised Homer, stating that he did not banish the cause of fear in *The Iliad* but painted a vivid picture of men facing death over and over. Longinus mentioned that Homer "expressed the emotion magnificently by crushing words together." He was critical of Plato, declaring that he "...is often carried away by a sort of literary madness into crude, harsh metaphors or allegorical fustian."

My main goal in pursuing the English degree was to add texture to my writing. Longinus provided the most practical and informative ways to write prose. I learned much from him. By incorporating some of his suggestions into my writing, texture improved.

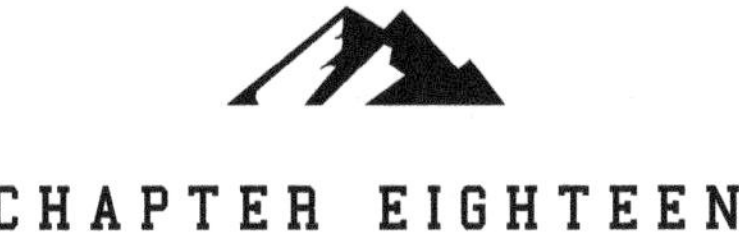

CHAPTER EIGHTEEN

Peers

"Don't try hard to fit in, and certainly don't try hard to be different...just try hard to be you."

— ZENDAYA

I spent six years in the company of my peers at York U., some for one semester, some for two semesters, and a few for three semesters. During that time, I observed them, scribbled notes about them, and tried to figure them out. I had attended university to pursue an English degree, the scholarly aspect of my learning; however, I had another kind of learning in mind all along—the social facet of my peers.

What did I, a retired person, a senior citizen, have in common with my peers, who were 99 percent millennials? We all came to York U. to learn academic information from the courses we took, to receive a passing grade, and finally, to obtain the prize—a degree in whatever field of endeavour each student chose. Those were perhaps the only things we had in common.

I learned a great deal about my peers, most young enough to be my grandchildren. Some of them were brilliant, some intelligent, and most were ambitious. They wanted to conquer the mountain and plant their flag on its summit. They hailed from various backgrounds and ethnicities—Indians, Chinese, Iranians, Jews, Africans, and West Indians, to name a few. They practiced all the major religions, based on their country of origin or that of their parents. The female Muslims stood out because many wore the hijab or headscarves at all times.

The mixture of ethnicity and culture created an interesting scenario. In one of my tutorials, after the professor asked several questions and received responses from the same handful of students, he proffered a question directly to a student wearing a hijab. She responded that she did not like to speak in class because she was quiet! Yet another student, also wearing a hijab, gave brilliant, articulate answers to questions in class. That incident reconfirmed what I'd learned over the years—it takes all types to make a world, and there is no complete homogeneity within cultures.

Canada was experiencing tough economic times in the early twenty-first century. It greatly impacted students. Many worked part-time to help pay their tuition fees and juggled their work time with university time. During lectures in the African American Literature class, Tallim, an Indian lad, usually sat beside me. We'd struck up a conversation, and I learned that he'd emigrated from Guyana and worked as a car mechanic. He was a handsome, pleasant fellow and one of the few students in the class who connected with me. I found it difficult to make any connection with most of my peers. They rarely looked you in the eye or initiated a conversation, and when I tried to engage them, they usually walked away. I think that most of them had no idea I was a senior citizen, although I thought I'd shown my age by never being seen talking on a cell phone and never arriving at classes with a laptop. They probably thought I carried it in my backpack, but I didn't own one then.

For tutorials, the tables were arranged in a square. One day, Tallim and I sat on the left side of the room near the back. The text for the class that day was by Olaudah Equiano, a twenty-five-page excerpt from his autobiography printed in *The Norton Anthology of African American Literature*. Professor Alston stood at the lectern at the front right corner of the room. She was speaking passionately about Equiano when Tallim let out a snore that sounded like an old train speeding into a rickety station. I quickly elbowed him in the ribs.

"Wake up! You can't sleep in class," I said, lowering my voice.

He opened his bloodshot eyes and looked at me. "Sorry, I'm tired. I had to work last night," he whispered.

The professor had not noticed our little sideshow, for she continued the lecture without glancing over at us. I felt compassion not only for Tallim, but for all the other students who had to rush from classes to work, then home. They were making sacrifices to obtain an education that would help them acquire better jobs, better incomes, and eventually, better futures. The incident brought me back to my first class, when Professor Blazina became angry that some students kept sending and receiving text messages during his lecture and not paying attention. There was a dichotomy of behaviours among my peers; some cared and made sacrifices, while others didn't care and just went along for the ride.

It didn't matter whether my peers were males or females, black, brown, or white: they wanted grades better than a C. I say bravo to them, provided they do the work. In one of my humanities classes, The Caribbean and Canada: Culture, Identity, and Diaspora, I noticed that more than half of the class were black students. It was my only course with such a high percentage of black students. Two professors taught the classes—one covered lectures, the other tutorials. The professor who taught tutorials gave us the assignment to write a research essay. I spent an inordinate amount of time searching online databases until I found the perfect articles to support my thesis. I wrote an essay that I thought was well written—by then, I was very confident writing essays.

The professor returned our marked essays at the end of one of our classes, just before lunchtime. I had made friends with Kayla, an attractive, plump black girl who usually sat in the row in front of me. She'd told me she was a single mother raising a four-year-old daughter. As soon as we received our essays, we gathered up our backpacks and walked together toward the food court. Kayla stopped to look at her mark and reacted furiously.

"Look at this. That woman gave me a D. I will not accept it."

"Kayla," I said, "before you get all worked up and say things to the professor that you shouldn't, let's look over the essay together."

She agreed. The food court was partially full when we arrived. We found a table away from the crowd and sat quietly. I pulled out my essay. My mark was B+.

"Okay, Kayla, let us compare oranges to oranges and see realistically if your essay deserved a better grade. I'll read my essay to you first, then you read yours, and we'll take it from there."

Kayla had accepted me as a mother figure and willingly listened to me. As I read my essay, the expression on her face told me she was impressed.

"Prof should have given you an A for that essay," she said when I completed the reading.

"An A would mean it's perfect. I'm happy with the B+."

Kayla read her essay. I would have drawn several red circles in it if I'd had a hard copy. The paragraphs had no connections. She made bold statements but had not supported her argument for the thesis with research articles. Even when she attempted to do so, it was not convincing. Her conclusion brought in new information and did not wrap up the essay well.

"Now that we've both read our essays, what do you think about your mark?" I asked.

Kayla looked at me, shamefaced. "I won't bother to approach the prof."

"I'm sorry to say this, Kayla, but you did a poor job with the essay. I know you could do better. What happened?"

She confessed that her daughter had been ill, and she had not spent much time working on the essay.

I empathized with her. "I truly admire you, Kayla. You are a single mother with a small child to take care of, yet you haven't given up on obtaining a degree. Keep going no matter the obstacles you come upon. Ask for help if you need it, but get that degree, then celebrate."

"Thank you, Mom," she said, laughing.

We clinked our bottles of juice together, then ate our lunches.

* * *

After I signed up for Law and Morality in Literature, I slipped away to Jamaica to spend a couple of weeks with a friend in St. Ann's Bay. The gorgeous sunshine, picturesque turquoise sea, fine white sand beaches, and exotic tropical fruits were just what I needed after a long, dreary winter. I hated to miss a class and had only missed two. This time, before I returned from Jamaica, the two first classes would have occurred.

The contact information for all class participants was available on the course's website. On my return to Toronto, I emailed one of my classmates requesting a copy of notes she had taken during the two classes I'd missed. The classmate never replied. When I attended class the following Tuesday, I asked a male student who sat next to me in the lecture theatre to send me a copy of his notes for the first two lectures. He agreed, and I wrote my email address on his notepad. He never sent his notes either. What was so hard about a classmate helping out another by sharing notes? Was it selfishness? Did he think, "My notes are for me and me alone?" Whatever the reason for the unhelpful behaviour of my classmates, I could not condone it or behave that way.

Law and Morality in Literature was a six-credit course. At the midpoint of the second semester, Jeff, a skinny, brown-haired student with a goatee and glasses, came over to me in the lecture hall during a short break. He was one of three students in the class of more than one hundred who spoke to me.

"Hi, Yvonne, I would like to ask you a favour," Jeff said, looking sheepish.

I looked up at him and smiled. “Sure, what is it?”

“I’m going away on a retreat, and I’m going to miss two classes. I know you take copious notes.” He laughed and looked away briefly. “Can you share your notes for the two classes with me when I return?”

“No problem, it will be my pleasure. I’ll email the notes to you after I type them up,” I promised Jeff. The mere idea that he noticed my avid notetaking made him good enough to share my notes.

I always took notes in class in longhand. I wrote and wrote until my wrist hurt. I have a stack of notebooks to prove it. It’s a small wonder that I didn’t develop carpal tunnel syndrome. Arriving at home after each class, I usually typed the notes on my desktop computer, printed a copy, and placed it in a file for my reviews. Having a memory that had lost some sharpness, interacting with my notes twice during a short time frame was an effective way to retain the information.

As I typed the notes from the lectures on Law and Morality in Literature, I was extra careful with my grammar and spelling, determined that none of my peers should find fault with my work. The two classes that Jeff missed were lectures on “The Roman Empire and The Rise of the Catholic Church.” The professor discussed Martin Luther and his criticism of the Catholic Church when it tried to finance the building of St. Peter’s Basilica by selling indulgences, and his criticism of rulers. I emailed perfect notes to Jeff. I was pleased to share them, knowing I’d helped a fellow student to get caught up with his lessons. He would not have to worry about missing valuable information before the exam. Jeff showed great appreciation for the notes and gave me a Tim Hortons card. I naturally told him there was no need for it, but he would not back down, so I took it. Weeks later, I took the card to the coffee shop, expecting it to be worth five dollars. I discovered it was worth twenty dollars. “Oh, Jeff, you shouldn’t have,” I thought, but alas! It was too late. Classes had ended, and Jeff and I had moved on to other courses. We never saw each other again.

It was no secret that many students had debts. Many had obtained student loans to finance their studies, since some parents could not cover tuition and book expenses. Student debt had been a constant issue in the media, but I was shocked when the actual numbers glared at me. I was walking through Vari Hall, heading toward the West Accolade building one day, when I observed that sections of the wall were covered with hundreds of strips of white construction paper with bold black numbers written on them. I stopped to investigate what the display was. The caption above the strips of paper read, "My student debt." My curiosity soared immediately. I moved from wall to wall, reading the numbers. The dollar figures of the debts included $40K, $50K, $70K, $20K, $5K, even a few $100K. Eight or nine strips had "$0" written on them. When I saw figures above $50K, I wondered, How on earth could a student owe so much money before starting out in the working world? How would they manage those debts if they had to live on their own after graduation?

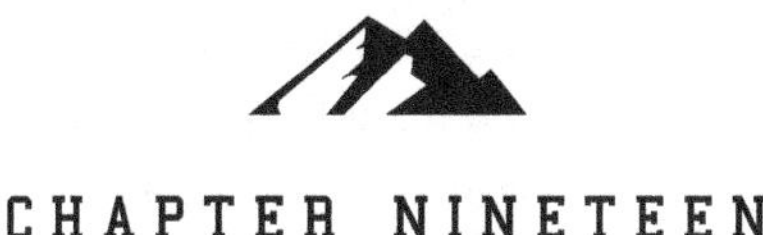

CHAPTER NINETEEN

Lessons on Environmental Pollution

"Knowledge is power. Information is liberating. Education is the premise of progress, in every society, in every family."

—KOFI ANNAN

Edging closer and closer to the finish line, excited, I pressed toward the mark for the prize. I checked the Academic Calendar for the Faculty of Liberal Arts & Professional Studies again to see if any mandatory courses were outstanding. Yes, I still needed three credits to fulfill the natural science requirement. I searched the NATS site and perused the courses offered in the fall semester of 2020. And there, blinking at me like a firefly in a dark night, was the course Environmental Pollution.

I had long believed that air and water pollution caused some of the cancers in our society, but no one was shouting it from the rooftops. Perhaps this course would shed light on the subject. Climate change had become very topical. It was on the lips of many people.

Actions on climate change strengthened with the adoption of the Kyoto Protocol in 1997. People began to pay significantly more attention when Al Gore, former vice president of the United States, debuted his film *An Inconvenient Truth* in 2006. In August 2018, Swedish climate activist Greta Thunberg protested in front of the Swedish Parliament, raising awareness for global warming and this spurred more awareness.

I considered the options for my final natural science course. What better time to learn the truth about pollution from the best authority—scientists—instead of the news? I registered for Environmental Pollution. The course outline stated that we would examine pollution with a focus on air, water, and soil pollution. The textbook for the course, *Understanding Environmental Pollution*, was written by Marquita K. Hill. She had been a scholar in environmental health at Harvard School of Public Health for seven years. I figured she would know the absolute truth about pollution.

Great.

I expected to learn much and confirm my belief that air and water pollution caused some cancers.

All of the courses at York U. remained online since March. I still didn't like that delivery method; however, Professor Dominikos taught her class in a way that made it more engaging than the one and a half courses I'd done online so far. My classes were on Mondays and Fridays from 1:00 p.m. to 2:20 p.m. The lectures were via Zoom, and students could use the chat box to ask questions during the class. The professor paused her talk and responded immediately to most questions. That way, I felt more involved in the class. I could read the questions my classmates asked and the answers given right there on the screen. She also recorded and posted all lectures. If you missed a Zoom class during the scheduled time, you could listen to the recording later on.

First, Professor Dominikos gave the class a quick quiz, a myth buster, to ascertain what we knew or believed about pollution. The responses surprised her and also me. Many students knew little about the problems caused by environmental pollution. I concluded that they needed the course as much as I did.

We delved into the course by first exploring air pollution. Since we would study the three main types of pollutants, I immediately thought of three questions I wanted answered: What were the primary pollutants? What were the sources of these pollutants? What were the main effects on humans and the environment of these pollutants? The class did not only read passages from the textbook; the professor applied her scientific knowledge to answer these questions in her lectures.

We learned that the five highest air pollutants that affect our health are: carbon monoxide; nitrogen oxides; sulphur dioxide; ground-level ozone; and particulate matter. These pollutants, termed criteria air pollutants (CAPs), are regulated by the World Health Organization (WHO). The professor mentioned that the Environmental Protection Agency (EPA) considers ozone (a large part of smog) the most dangerous and persistent air quality problem in the United States. Similar to Understanding Food, the other natural science course I had taken, I was required to learn a few scientific formulas that included the five primary pollutants.

My informed professor explained that worldwide, 90 percent of the energy powering the turbines that produce electricity comes from burning fossil fuels—coal, oil, and natural gas. Burning coal discharges sulphur, carbon monoxide, nitrogen oxides, and particulate matter into the air. Burning natural gas releases carbon monoxide and nitrogen oxides. Burning gasoline for vehicles releases carbon monoxide, nitrogen oxides, and particulate matter into the air. Combustion of these fossil fuels also discharges CO2 and contributes to the greenhouse gases that cause 75 percent of the present warming of the earth. Ozone is a secondary pollutant created by chemical reactions in the atmosphere. Particulate matter is solid particles like soot and soil dust. In addition to burning fossil fuels, forest fires, lightning, and volcanoes deposit sulphur, carbon monoxide, and nitrogen oxides into the air.

What is the effect of air pollution on humans? The goodly professor answered the question this way:

> According to the WHO, air pollution accounts for:
> 29% of all deaths and diseases from lung cancer
> 17% of all deaths and diseases from an acute lower respiratory infection
> 25% of all deaths from strokes
> 25% of all deaths and diseases from coronary heart disease
> 43% of all deaths and diseases from chronic obstructive pulmonary disease (COPD)

Professor Dominikos explained that particulate matter and ground-level ozone enter our bodies through our noses and mouths. Particulate matter causes asthma, chronic bronchitis, and heart attacks. Ozone causes lung and throat irritation, coughing, shortness of breath, and reduced lung function, and aggravates asthma and chronic lung disease.

I was keen to learn about the ozone, another topical subject in the news. Where was it? What purpose did it serve? Our scientific professor gave us the facts: 90 percent of all ozone molecules in the atmosphere are in the stratosphere. Ground-level ozone harms humans; however, those same ozone molecules in the stratosphere protect humans and the earth from harmful ultraviolet (UV) radiation. The information blew me away. Suddenly, ozone was not the mysterious thing I had thought. It was comforting to have dangerous subjects explained in simple terms.

We studied the different types of ultraviolet radiation and the baffling ozone hole. Once again, we learned that human activity is the primary cause of the destruction of the ozone. In 1928, a chemist developed a new coolant called chlorofluorocarbon (CFC), and in 1950, another scientist developed a chemical called halon. When these two chemicals entered the stratosphere and interacted with ultraviolet light, they caused the gradual destruction of the ozone. The information I learned about air pollution was scary but fascinating.

Professor Dominikos gave us a test at the end of the air pollution segment. I taxed my brain cells and crammed for it more than I had done for any other class. I believe knowing air pollution affected me personally caused the information to stick. I received 93 percent on the test.

In the middle of the semester, Professor Dominikos dived into the subject of water pollution. I had many misconceptions about this topic, and this segment was just as illuminating as the one about air pollution. First, she defined water pollution as: "The contamination of bodies of water (such as lakes, rivers, oceans, groundwater etc.) when pollutants are directly or indirectly discharged into them without adequate treatment." She explained that pollution into a single lake does not necessarily stay there permanently. The water cycle connects the atmosphere to water reservoirs, which include lakes, oceans, groundwater, springs, snow, glaciers, permafrost, wetlands, plants, and animals. Water moves *to* the atmosphere via evaporation—water to gas or vapour; sublimation—ice and snow change from solid to liquid; and evapotranspiration—evaporated water from plants and soils. The reverse process transports water *from* the atmosphere by condensation—gas to liquid; precipitation—rain, snow, hail; deposition—gas to solid. As a result of the water cycle process, contaminated water moves around.

What were the primary water pollutants?

The six primary water pollutants that are often present in large amounts are:

Biochemical oxygen demand—not enough oxygen to decompose organic material.

Nutrients—too much nitrogen and phosphorous enter the water systems. It could come from runoff of fertilizer from fields, animal manure, sewage and wastewater, and laundry detergents and soaps.

Suspended soil—soil tossed about by the wind.

PH level—the acidity or alkaline level in the water.

Oil and grease—runoff from asphalt and oil spills.

Pathogenic microorganisms—a pathogen, a bacterium, virus, fungus, protozoan and toxic algal species enter the water cycle.

What were the main effects of these pollutants on humans and the environment?

Professor Dominikos explained how the six water pollutants affect the environment:

Nutrients can degrade the ecosystem by causing algae near the water surface to grow fast and block the sun from marine animals and plants below. Eventually, the algae die, sink to the bottom, and become food for decomposers. As they break down the algae, they remove oxygen from the water, limiting oxygen to fish and plants.

Oil is less dense than water, so it floats on the surface and affects the ecosystem. The main impact is: oil destroys the insulating ability of fur-bearing mammals like otters and decreases the water-repelling of birds' feathers. Birds and mammals die from hypothermia when they cannot repel water and insulate themselves from cold. Also, many water creatures come up to the surface for oxygen. If they inhale oil, it affects their lungs, immune function, and reproduction. Oil spills block the sunlight marine plants need to photosynthesize, killing plants growing in the water. We were surprised to learn that despite several large oil spills by tankers over the years, they are a minor contributor to the oil found in oceans. Fifty percent of oil currently found in oceans come from land-based sources like asphalt runoff, offshore discharges, and oil transporting and shipping.

PH levels in water should not be too acidic or too alkaline. It is the most common pollutant in rivers, streams, and lakes. The PH level is most important to marine life, and if disturbed enough could kill marine animals.

Suspended soil occurs from mining, construction, and land clearing. When humans remove vegetation, the soil becomes exposed to wind and water transport. The EPA lists suspended soil as the most common pollutant in rivers, streams, lakes, and reservoirs. Sediment can clog the gills of fishes, reduce their resistance to disease, and lower their growth rates. Suspended soil can alter the water flow, reduce water depth, and affect navigation. It can fill up storm drains and catch basins and increase the potential for flooding.

The main pathogenic microorganisms usually present in bacterially polluted waters can cause several diseases. Bacteria can cause cholera and typhoid fever; viruses can cause poliomyelitis and hepatitis. Helminth can cause tapeworms. Bacteria in water also affect coral. The coral of the Great Barrier Reef was dramatically affected by bacteria.

Water pollution and plastics are subjects lately discussed ad nauseam. Professor Dominikos enlightened us on the topic: Plastic waste does not decompose readily, and large amounts remain in the environment for a long time. Some studies on plastics suggest that it takes thousands of years to decompose plastic bags and Styrofoam containers. Globally, only 9 percent of more than nine billion tonnes of plastic produced is recycled. Studies estimate that seven million tonnes of the world's plastics end up in the oceans yearly.

The professor gave us the assignment to research the Great Pacific Garbage Patch. We also watched a film about it. I learned a lot from the exercise. The information gathered allowed me to understand that not only do plastics directly pose a physical threat to wildlife, but they also pose a chemical threat to humans.

For the final stretch of Environmental Pollution, we examined soil pollution. Professor Dominikos defined it as: "The presence of a chemical or substance out of place and/or present at a higher-than-normal concentration that has adverse effects on any non-target organism." The Food and Agriculture Organization of the United Nations estimates that twenty-two million hectares of land globally are affected by soil pollution.

I had never paid much attention to soil pollution, but I quickly learned it was almost as important as air and water.

My informed professor listed the main culprits and elaborated on what they are:

Heavy metals and metalloids
Nitrogen and phosphorus
Pesticides
Persistent organic pollutants (POPs)
Radionuclides
Emerging pollutants

Heavy metals include lead, cadmium, copper, mercury, tin, and zinc. The primary sources of these metals come from coal plants (mercury), paints, leaded gasoline, mining, and smelting. Heavy metals are the most persistent and complex pollutants to remove from the environment.

What were the primary effects of these pollutants on humans and the environment?

Mercury is toxic to the human central and peripheral nervous systems. It can cause tremors, insomnia, memory loss, and cognitive and motor dysfunction. Lead can cause anemia, weakness, kidney and brain damage, and nervous system damage. Cadmium can affect kidneys and cause bone and lung disease.

Pesticides include insecticides, fungicides, and herbicides. Pesticides are used for good reasons. They help crops grow year-round; crops can grow in inappropriate regions; they kill disease-carrying organisms; food can be stored longer; and they help the aesthetics of some foods. But pesticides can affect humans by causing cancer and harm to developing fetuses or small children. It can also affect non-target species; it kills birds, fish, amphibians, and pollinating insects.

Persistent organic pollutants (POPs) are organic chemical substances with a particular combination of physical and chemical properties. They include pesticides, polychlorinated biphenyl (PCB), and dioxin. When these substances get released into the atmosphere, they remain there for long periods. They naturally become distributed widely throughout the environment by soil, air, and water. The health effect is these substances accumulate in fatty tissues of living organisms and are toxic to humans and wildlife.

Radionuclides are created naturally from cosmic radiation and by humans from the fallout from atmospheric nuclear weapons testing, operations of nuclear facilities, and nuclear accidents. Radionuclides travel in the environment through the air and water and get deposited in the soil. Plants take it up in their roots, and it eventually enters the food chain. After the Chernobyl nuclear accident, there was a significant increase in leukemia and thyroid cancer in young children and adolescents.

Emerging pollutants are several synthetic or naturally occurring chemicals that have recently appeared in the environment. Currently, no one monitors them regularly, but scientists believe they harm the environment and humans. These chemicals include pharmaceutical and personal care products (PPCPs), endocrine disruptors, and biological pollutants. These products enter urban wastewater streams, but conventional treatment technologies do not efficiently eliminate them. They end up in sludge that is applied to land as fertilizer. Endocrine disruptors are plasticizers added to plastic and other products to make them more flexible. These chemicals mimic the natural hormone estrogen. Like PPCPs, they are not effectively removed from sludge applied to agricultural fields and can cause contamination. Both PPCPs and endocrine disruptors have been detected in food and humans.

Environmental Pollution did not disappoint. Professor Dominikos answered my three questions about each type of pollution in simple terms. She added some case locations and incidents that occurred in recent times that made the learning more meaningful. You may be asking if my long-time belief that some cancers in our society are caused by environmental pollution was addressed. Yes, 110 percent. The sad thing is that pollution not only causes some cancers, it causes a myriad of other diseases too. I feel much better informed about our world, and I encourage my fellow seniors to take at least one course on the subject.

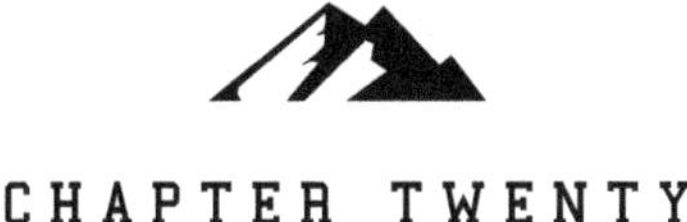

CHAPTER TWENTY

My World Stood Still

"Bad news isn't wine. It doesn't improve with age."
—COLIN POWELL

Back in 2018, I became convinced that the stars were not aligned in my favour to achieve my goal of obtaining an English degree by my seventieth birthday. The long-drawn-out strike at York U. had seen to that. The strike ended on July 25th, and I was forging ahead when COVID-19 struck, and all courses moved online from March 2020. It meant that I had to accept doing classes online, for nothing would stop me from succeeding. I shifted my graduation date to 2021. I had no inkling that something worse than COVID-19 lurked in the shadows.

* * *

The phone at home rang one Sunday morning in early December 2020. The number on the display screen looked unfamiliar. I usually do not answer calls from unknown numbers, but a small voice in my head said, "Answer it." I did. The person on the line identified himself as a doctor from Mt. Sinai Hospital. Surprised, I said, "I didn't know doctors worked on Sundays." He replied that he was backed up with patients and had decided to make a few Sunday calls. After that, he said he had reviewed my MRI, ultrasound, and biopsy reports. I had done these procedures about a month earlier after I found a lump on my right thigh.

The doctor said that the lump was sarcoma cancer.

The earth stood still.

My heart stopped beating.

The air in the room evaporated.

It felt like I had clicked the "shutdown" button on my computer, and the bright, colourful icons disappeared, leaving the screen black as midnight. Several of my friends and colleagues had contracted or succumbed to the dreadful disease called cancer. We ate the same foods, drank water from the same source, and breathed the same air. Cancer had finally caught up with me; I suppose it was only a matter of time before I received such a diagnosis.

It seemed like a lifetime before I found my voice.

"What is that? I've never heard of sarcoma," I said.

The doctor explained that sarcoma is a type of cancer that can occur in various parts in your body. There are more than seventy types, and it usually attacks the soft tissue, like muscles, and tends to be localized.

The earth began to revolve again.

My breathing resumed.

My heartbeat normalized.

"How is it cured?" I asked.

"Treatment is usually radiation and surgery. Sometimes patients receive radiation first, then surgery, or vice versa," the doctor said. He mentioned that the MRI I had done earlier was not very clear, and it appeared there might be more than one tumour in my thigh. He planned to order another MRI, biopsy, and CT scan for me before he did anything. I thanked him for wanting to be so thorough and waited for the new appointment dates.

I had been on the board of the College of Nurses for several years and learned much about the Health Colleges of Ontario. I knew that the College of Physicians and Surgeons is the regulatory body for doctors and physicians who have a license to practice in the province and must register with this organization. If there were complaints or disciplinary actions against a doctor, the college recorded them on its website. After I hung up, I searched the CPS site for information on the doctor. It turned out that the doctor was a sarcoma specialist, and his record was clean as a new cotton ball.

The Internet provides tons of information, but one must be careful to access it only from reputable sites. My go-to site for health and medical information is the Mayo Clinic. I searched their site. It confirmed everything the doctor told me about sarcoma and provided more details.

* * *

I needed to earn nine credits to complete my degree. *Tentanda via.* Despite the cancer diagnosis, I remained resolute that I would continue my studies. Assuming it would take months before I did the new tests the doctor prescribed and he took any action, I registered for the three-credit course 20th Century Children's Literature, scheduled to start in early January. The course outline stated it would examine three main elements of children's literature from the twentieth and twenty-first centuries: the literature, the children, and the adult critics.

All of York U.'s courses remained online because COVID-19 refused to disappear. The professor posted the syllabus on the university's site and listed sixteen books required for the class. They consisted of picture books, chapbooks, and young adult books, including *Harriet the Spy*, *Harry Potter and the Philosopher's Stone,* and *The Hunger Games*. In addition, students had to read several theoretical papers that examined the definition of children's literature, concerns about the construction of children, and the issue of power and childhood. "Whoa, this course is not simply about reading fairy tales," I thought.

The first lecture tackled Beatrix Potter's *The Tale of Peter Rabbit,* published in 1902. I'd read some of the Peter Rabbit adventures many moons ago and thought he was a cute, lovable bunny (the pastel-coloured pictures in the books certainly were); I considered it a good story for children. Now, here we were, 119 years later, scrutinizing the text and illustrations and discovering that Peter, the only boy rabbit in the family, was subversive, defiant, disobedient, and adventurous. But his three sisters were "Good little bunnies," obedient and unadventurous. In essence, Peter presented a bad influence on children.

Next, we explored two Winnie-the-Pooh stories. They were exciting as I viewed them through a newer, clearer lens. Written by A. A. Milne, and published in 1926 and 1928, *Winnie- the-Pooh* and *The House at Pooh Corner* helped me grasp the author's nostalgia and longing for the idyll of prewar years and the lush English countryside. Christopher Robin was the only human in the stories, and he lived among a cast of animals, including his best friend, Winnie-the-Pooh, in and around the lush, green Hundred Acre Wood. A pristine stream ran through the land, and the characters played pop-stick from a bridge built over it. Everyone worked together and helped each other except Eeyore, the donkey. He constantly complained but eventually changed and became more accommodating. The stories showed the importance of friendships and working together. They are positive for children.

The text that captured my attention the most was *Harriet the Spy.* The novel was published in 1964, and said to have introduced the New Realism to children's literature. It eliminated mannerly, polite children and the sugarcoated behaviours of parents. Harriet spied on the people in her neighbourhood. She knew their dirty little secrets and wrote about them in her diary. The novel highlighted children's emotions and subversive imaginations. It alarmed many parents. The 20th Century Children's Literature course certainly opened my eyes to the subtleties of children's literature. It taught me not to take children's stories at face value. You should consider the history and geography of the times they were written.

After the doctor reviewed the final tests and confirmed that I definitely had sarcoma cancer, I shared the information with friends and family. Several people offered up prayers for me. My church family, my Caribbean posse ladies, my close friends, and family members all became part of the prayer group. Prayers worked.

I was on the final stretch of the course with four weeks remaining when I received a call from a radiologist at Princess Margaret hospital. I'd met him along with the sarcoma specialist a few weeks earlier. He called to say that my radiation treatments would begin on March 15th. He reminded me that treatments would last five weeks, and I would receive them five days each week, Mondays to Fridays.

"I'm doing a course at York University, and I don't want to withdraw from it. Will I be okay to continue my studies while receiving radiation treatments?" I asked.

"Radiation will not affect your brain," he said. We both laughed. "You can continue your studies."

Thinking about the timing of the treatments, I realized that it would be a problem for me. The Princess Margaret hospital stood smack in the heart of downtown Toronto, and I lived about sixty kilometres north in Richmond Hill. I would not drive downtown for treatment. It would be physically difficult for me to travel back and forth. I could not in good conscience expect my son to take me five days per week for the treatments; he worked and had two young sons to care for. I also felt it would be too burdensome on two girlfriends, who had already driven me to several doctor's appointments, to ask them to take me. I concluded that my best option would be to live at a hotel near the hospital for the five weeks.

Gloria, one of my Caribbean posse ladies, took me to meet her friend, Edith, a retired doctor. Dr. Edith offered to accommodate me in her beautiful Rosedale home for the duration of my treatment. She also volunteered her husband, Michael, to drive me to and from the hospital every treatment day, provided my appointments were after 11:00 a.m. I had no say in setting appointment times. The hospital assigned the appointment times based on the number of patients requiring treatment and the personnel available. As luck would have it (or was it prayers answered?), the hospital scheduled mine for noon and some for 1:00 p.m. Michael became my chauffeur for five weeks.

Once I finalized the accommodation arrangements with Dr. Edith, I phoned Ross, my former senior classmate who knew a lot about computers, to recommend a laptop I should purchase. He suggested a Dell, and I bought one. It was a sleek little device, thin, lightweight, and fast. I wondered why I hadn't bought one before. Then I remembered that I'd stuck with a desktop computer because the adjustable monitor and keyboard allowed me to sit back in my office chair without straining my back and neck. I took the laptop with me to my temporary Rosedale home, so I could continue my studies while receiving radiation treatments.

My accommodation at Dr. Edith's home was luxurious, to put it mildly. My suite, located at the west wing of the house, was furnished with a gorgeous mahogany four-poster, queen-sized bed, the posts skillfully crafted with pineapple designs. The only thing missing was the canopy! My host strategically placed two desks in the room, one near a window and the other near the bed. A chaise lounge stood at the foot of the bed. The large closets had mirrored doors; the floors were pristine hardwood. Vertical blinds covered a bank of windows that looked out onto the street. I opened them every morning as soon as the sun came up. Across the street was a park with several permanent benches. Walking trails meandered through the park, and the residents took full advantage of them. Looking out the windows, I could see snippets of the Don Valley Parkway in the distance. Once I ascended the stairs to my suite, I neither saw nor heard anyone; the peace was just what I needed.

Dr. Edith was a real-life angel who took me under her wing. She was petite, with a thick head of hair that she covered with a hairnet. She spoke softly, enunciating every word. The first morning I came downstairs for breakfast, she served me on a tray in the living room. The second morning, as she placed the breakfast tray on a side table, she looked directly into my eyes and asked, "Do you not take supplements, Yvonne?"

Surprised at the question, I stuttered, “Yes…, but I didn’t bring any with me. I take them inconsistently, anyway. I guess it’s the rebel in me.”

The truth was, I purchased supplements often but never took them regularly and usually had to throw some out because the dates expired.

“You need to take supplements,” she said emphatically.

The next morning, she placed a small pill cup with four pills on my breakfast tray: vitamins D3, B12, and B100, plus calcium. For the five weeks I lived in Dr. Edith’s home, she placed the pill cup with four pills on my breakfast tray every morning.

* * *

On the first day of radiation treatment in March, I arrived at Princess Margaret hospital wearing a skirt and a blouse, a light spring coat, and a mask. It mattered not whether you came with or without a mask because the attendants at the door gave you a fresh one before they allowed you to step onto the hospital floor because of COVID-19. Sitting in the waiting room in the treatment centre, socially distanced from other patients, I felt afraid. What would radiation treatment be like? How long would each session take? Would I feel sick afterward? A female technician pushed open a large door and stepped into the waiting room. She called my name. I responded, “Over here,” and walked toward her. She greeted me pleasantly and escorted me to a chair in the hallway. She inquired how I felt. Observing my skirt, she said I did not need to change into a gown. She led me into a room with a gigantic machine, one bigger than any CAT scan or MRI machine I had seen. It had arms that revolved, and a bed. Another female technician in the room greeted me. I removed my coat and shoes, and both technicians helped me onto the bed. Before lying down, I explained that there was a bulging disk in my lower back, and if I lay flat for a few minutes, I would be in pain.

The ladies quickly produced pillows and a little cradle to support my back. I lay down and felt comfortable. They spent ten minutes putting on the plastic mould made for my right leg two weeks earlier and positioning me for the laser treatment that had to be precise. They checked and cross-checked, and recorded measurements. One technician instructed me not to move my right leg during treatment. They had strapped it down anyway. I could not move it if I tried.

When the technicians felt everything was in order, one asked, "Are you comfortable, Mrs. Blackwood?"

"Yes, I am," I replied.

"Would you like some music?"

"Music? What kind do you have?"

"Oh, we have a variety. Simon and Garfunkel, Bob Marley—"

"Stop right there, play Bob Marley," I said.

She laughed and inserted a disc into a small boom box on a shelf on the left side of the room. She pressed play, then turned on the huge radiation machine. Both technicians left the room at that point.

I lay back on the bed and watched the lights flicker and the machine perform its movements. I closed my eyes and said a prayer. I prayed to the good Lord that the radiation would accomplish what the doctors expected and that I wouldn't suffer any side effects. At that moment, I felt that God was in the room with me. Absolute peace swept over me. Bob Marley's voice filtered throughout the room, singing:

> Don't worry, about a thing
> 'Cause every little thing, gonna be all right
> Singin', don't worry, about a thing
> 'Cause every little thing, gonna be all right.

I opened my eyes and looked around. I thought this must surely be a sign that I was going to be okay. The song seemed so apropos, so profound, so reassuring. "Three Little Birds" was the fourth song on Bob Marley's *Legend*, one of my favourite albums. It begins with those words. Why had the music started with that particular song and those specific words? I sang along with the chorus and counted on my fingers the number of zaps each tumour received. The actual treatment lasted about fifteen minutes, or four Bob Marley songs.

The technicians repeated the same procedure for the remaining twenty-four treatments, but shortened their set-up time as they became more proficient. They played Bob Marley discs for me every day, and every day, I sang along. Each day I left the treatment room feeling upbeat and healthy. The technicians must have been watching me through a concealed window because, on the third day, one asked me if I had been counting during treatment.

Michael drove me directly home to Rosedale after each radiation treatment. My energy was zapped. Dr. Edith offered me a cappuccino as soon as I stepped through the front door. She insisted I sit in the reclining chair and put my feet up.

"Your feet must be higher than your bum," she advised.

Later in the evening, she persuaded me to take a walk with her and Michael, and we did this several times. Dr. Edith and Michael were not only avid readers, but they were also keen movie watchers. They encouraged me to join them in the family room in the basement on Thursdays for movie nights. Dr. Edith would come down to the family room carrying a tray loaded with tea and goodies she had baked, and we enjoyed them while watching the movie selected by one of us.

I believe she adopted me!

Every day, after enjoying delicious cappuccinos, I took naps, logged into the York U. website, and joined the Zoom lectures. While I lived at Dr. Edith's, I read five novels and two PDF academic articles relating to children's literature, and completed and submitted the last quiz on time.

* * *

The politicians announced the COVID-19 vaccine rollout to Ontarians. To receive it, they merely had to register.

The first group to receive the vaccine between December 2020 and March 2021 were:

Congregate living for seniors
Health care workers
Adults in First Nations, Métis and Inuit populations
Adult chronic home care recipients
Adults aged 80 and older

The second group scheduled for the vaccine between April and June 2021 were adults aged fifty-five and older. I was residing at Dr. Edith's home when my age group received the green light to obtain the shot. She went online, found a clinic several kilometres from her home, and registered herself and Michael. The kind soul probably thought I wouldn't have time or patience to go through the registration process based on the difficulty she had experienced. The next day, she trotted up the stairs to my suite and knocked on the door. She intended to register me for the shot. Would I provide her with my health card information? I gladly gave it to her. I'd quickly learned that when Dr. Edith had an idea, she became like a dog with a bone. She does not stop until she achieves what she has set out to do.

Dr. Edith spent two hours online, getting kicked out and going back in, until she completed the registration for me, and one of her friends. She heard that the clinic would provide the vaccine even if you were a few days short of the deadline, and I was. On March 30th, Michael drove me and Dr. Edith's friend to the vaccination clinic, where we received our first shots. I felt a bit safer. I remain eternally grateful to Dr. Edith and Michael.

* * *

I believe that if there is a time of year to be ill and confined to the house during a raging pandemic, it is springtime. When your spirits are topsy-turvy, and you are wondering what radiation treatments are doing to your body, nothing offers as much uplifting feeling or healing power as Mother Nature. Standing at my Rosedale bedroom window, I watched the trees reclothe in the park across the street. Delicate green shoots developed rapidly until the area that once looked like a wilderness of dried sticks morphed into a forest of greenery. The view stimulated a calm and soothing feeling within me.

I observed bright yellow crocuses, the first spring flowers, appear in Dr. Edith's small garden at the front of the house. I watched a patch of blue *Scilla siberica*, bell-shaped flowers that look like tiny lilies, begin their blooming period one by one, and within two weeks, a ribbon of blue flowers had captured a strip of grass at the edge of the park.

One day, as Michael drove me home from the hospital, he deviated from the usual route and passed by a particular house at the corner of a street. I was awestruck by the view. The entire front lawn was a thick carpet of delicate blue. *Scilla siberica* plants had captured it. He parked the car close to the house, and I stepped out and took pictures. I posted one on Facebook, and it garnered several likes. I noticed that several magnolia trees in the neighbourhood had begun to flower, the buds taking their time to open.

On Fridays after each radiation treatment, Michael drove me home to Rosedale, where I slurped Dr. Edith's delicious cappuccinos, then gathered my clothes to be laundered, textbooks, and laptop, and placed them in my car. Our goodbyes were long and drawn out, but eventually, I drove to my home in Richmond Hill. I spent the weekends dusting the furniture, washing clothes, cooking enough for the weekend, and studying.

I looked forward to seeing my two young grandsons. Rob brought them over on Sundays. They would come charging through the front door like bulls at a bullfight. I stopped being fussy about keeping the house in order and allowed them to play in the long hallway, where at least they would avoid bumping into furniture. I kept a large, blue exercise ball in my bedroom upstairs, and Theo, the older one, would lug it downstairs, jump on it, and roll down the hallway. Anthony would jump on him, and for the next hour or so, both boys rode the ball up and down the hallway, squealing and having fun. No electronic device gave them so much pleasure. The squealing and laughter were loud, but I didn't mind the noise in the house. I was just grateful to see them and hug them.

Sunday evenings, I returned to Rosedale, repeated the treatment routine, and continued my studies. The final exam for 20th Century Children's Literature was scheduled for the weekend of April 19th. I buckled down and started to review and reread most of the textbooks.

The professor allocated our marks based on at least eight posts responding to her discussion questions and eight meaningful replies to our classmates' responses; two quizzes consisting of ten multiple-choice questions—one done in February and one in March; an essay in mid-March (I wrote this while undergoing radiation); and a ninety-minute final exam.

By the time my treatments ended mid-April, the crocuses in Dr. Edith's garden had withered, but the space was brimming with tulips and other colourful flowers. The magnolia trees in the area now exhibited magnificent blooms. The neighbourhood was a wonderland of colours and beauty, a breath of fresh air.

I returned home to Richmond Hill the Friday afternoon after my final radiation treatment. I spent most of Saturday and Sunday reviewing the lectures and my notes for the second half of the semester. I wrote my final exam on Monday.

I never informed the professor or my classmates about my illness or treatments.

Dr. Edith and Michael have remained good friends.

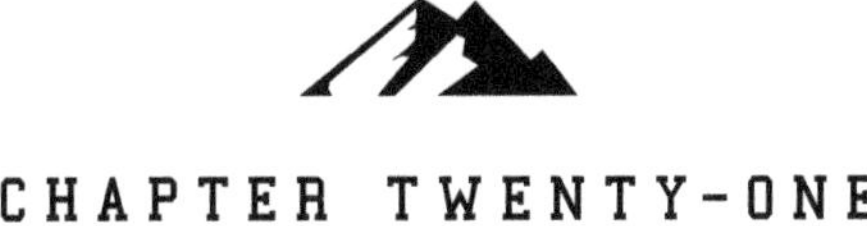

CHAPTER TWENTY-ONE

Hospital Room Classroom

"Nothing is impossible, the word itself says I'm possible!"
—AUDREY HEPBURN

I was happy to be back at my home, though I missed Dr. Edith and Michael. It had been a joy to banter with them as I ate breakfast in the mornings and listened to Michael read articles from the newspaper about current issues. Fatigue from the radiation treatment dissipated. I felt great. I walked out onto the deck to see what had become of the backyard and the regularly visiting fauna while I was away for the past five weeks. The weeds had grown as high as the shrubs, a phenomenon that always baffled me—weeds that grew faster than the plants we nurtured. The squirrels still jumped from branch to branch on the tall cedar trees that provided privacy for the backyard of the townhouse complex. But the sounds of the birds chirping—blue jays, cardinals, grackles, juncos, redwing blackbirds, robins, sparrows, yellow finches—were missing.

I stepped back inside the house, dashed upstairs, and looked out my bedroom window. I observed a flourish of wildlife activity in my neighbour's backyard to the right. It seemed they had created an aviary! Several birds gathered there, including a pair of mourning doves I had never before seen in the backyard. My neighbours had placed several bird feeders laden with seeds in various spots along their fence, and the birds were feasting. One lone bird feeder hung from my back fence—seedless, empty.

* * *

I resumed everyday life and turned my attention to my studies. I needed six lousy credits to earn my English degree. Who would be silly enough to give up at this stage? Who would wimp out when they were so close to the finish line? Who would forfeit the prize because of a shortfall of six credits? It would certainly not be me. I was determined to complete the task and refused to register for two three-credit courses. Only ONE six-credit course would do. I had fulfilled the requirements for social science, natural science, the humanities, and had already obtained the thirty-credit minimum required for the major in English.

Which course should I make my last hurrah? I had thoroughly enjoyed all the English classes. Why not register for another? I had published only adult nonfiction books but had begun writing a novel. Thinking that a creative writing course would provide additional ammunition for novel writing, I registered for the six-credit summer course Introduction to Creative Writing.

The overview stated:

> The purpose is to introduce students to writing poetry and fiction through the practices that comprise the writing lives of published authors. It is designed to familiarize students with literary traditions and the possibilities of these forms, to help them explore creative reading/writing/editing processes, and to discover and hone their talents.

This course seemed ideal to conclude my long, obstacle-laden journey, to complete my mountain climb, and reach the summit. My thinking was: If I had surgery in June (hopefully near the end of June), I would be halfway through the final course then. It meant working extra hard in the first half to obtain excellent marks. If I became ill during the second half and received lower marks, the combined score would earn me an average grade for the first time. It would lower my GPA slightly, but I would obtain my degree.

With the university under lockdown since the declaration of the COVID-19 pandemic, classes continued via Zoom. In the first class, the professor, who was in her mid-thirties, with long brown hair and glasses, talked about herself and her years of teaching the course. She then asked all students on the call to introduce themselves. It seemed the introductions were not enough for her. She then asked us to write an autobiography and email it to her by the next class three days later. The document had to be at least two pages and double-spaced. Two pages was a lot of information, I thought. She listed some of the things she wanted us to include.

I was not thrilled with the request. During my studies at York U., I had avoided giving details about myself to professors and students. Now, with my last course, my incognito persona would be blown to bits. Why did the professor feel she had to gather so many details about the students? I believed she was being inquisitive. But what the heck? I would never see her in person or have any contact with her. I wrote my autobiography by merely responding to the list of questions she posed:

Who are you? I am a retired person, a mother, and grandmother. Name some things you love to do? I love to travel and have done so extensively. Do you own any pets? I own no pets—no dog, cat, fish, or iguana. Have you published anything? I have published three adult nonfiction books, three children's picture books, and several short stories. Who is your favourite author? It is hard to choose a favourite author because I read several genres; however, I enjoyed the work of Maya Angelou for her diction and fascinating life stories;

Michael Ondaatje for his way with words and interesting stories; John Grisham for his ability to keep me on the edge of my seat. Why are you taking this course? I'm taking the course because I am writing a novel and feel that it would help enhance my fiction writing.

I omitted all information about my banking career.

* * *

When I first met with the surgeon after the cancer diagnosis, he informed me that surgery would probably be sometime in June and that he usually waited several weeks after radiation treatment before removing the radiated tumours.

The dreaded call came earlier than I'd expected. My surgeon informed me that he planned to do the surgery to remove the sarcoma tumours from my right thigh on May 27th. On a cool Thursday morning, Rob, my son, drove me to Mt. Sinai Hospital at 6:00 a.m., then departed. With COVID-19 still looming large, the hospital did not allow anyone to enter and wait with me. I sat in the waiting room with about eight other patients. They all looked as scared as I was. My tote bag rested on the floor beside me with the few items allowed. I had received an information sheet at the pre-op meeting a few days earlier that specified that the hospital would not be responsible for any stolen valuables. Knowing this, I instructed Rob to keep my laptop in his car and bring it when he was allowed to visit. I would be permitted only one visitor on the day after surgery.

* * *

When I came out of the anesthesia, the first person I saw was the anesthesiologist, a pleasant man of about forty. We'd met when he visited me before the surgery to explain the procedure. Looking at me with compassion, he assured me the operation went well. My surgeon had removed the thigh muscles with sarcoma tumours and inserted a metal post to help strengthen the thigh. In addition, a plastic surgeon removed a flap and implanted it in the incision, attaching the blood vessels and nerves. The flap would also help to strengthen the thigh.

"The surgery lasted thirteen hours," the anesthesiologist said.

"Thirteen hours? My surgeon said it would last about nine hours," I said.

"The plastic surgeon didn't take the flap from your shoulder as originally planned. She took it from the upper part of your leg."

"Oh, great, at least I don't have to worry about pain in my shoulder and pain in my thigh," I said.

He touched my arm gently, wished me well, and left my bedside. I don't remember much about the rest of the day. I slept a lot. The next evening, Rob, the only visitor allowed, came. I saw a worried look on his face and assured him I was all right. He brought my laptop, which I booted up the next day.

I spent the first few days in Mt. Sinai Hospital recovering and regaining my strength. My right leg was wrapped in a brace called a Zimmer that stretched from my groin to my ankle. Nurses taught me to walk using a walker.

A female hospital personnel staff visited on the third day and advised me that I would be sent to a rehab centre.

"Which one?" I asked.

"Maybe The Rehab Centre across the street, or Bridgepoint Health at Gerrard and Broadview."

Dr. Edith had told me to request St. John's Rehab, mentioning that it provided excellent care.

"What about St. John's?" I asked.

"There's no guarantee that they'll have a bed available, but I'll check," she said.

Two days later, she returned. "You will need to pack up your belongings. The patient transporters will come tomorrow, after breakfast, to take you to Bridgepoint. It's an affiliate rehab hospital."

And that was that! I had no further discussion with the woman and no say in where I would rehabilitate.

At 10:30 a.m. the next day, two buff young men arrived at my room with a stretcher. They grasped the sheet on my hospital bed and swung me onto the stretcher. They placed the tote bag with my belongings and laptop beside me, then steered the stretcher out of the room, into the elevator, and down to the ground level, where an ambulance-like vehicle awaited. The patient transporters secured the stretcher in the van; then one of them drove it like an ambulance on a call (without the sirens) to Bridgepoint Health hospital. At the admitting counter, one of the men presented papers from Mt. Sinai to the attendant, and within minutes, the stretcher pulled up at the nurses' station on the second floor. Directed by two nurses, the patient transporters repeated the previous procedure and swung me in the sheet from the stretcher onto my new hospital bed, secured behind striped, pastel-coloured curtains. They wished me well and departed.

What do you do when they send you to a rehab hospital where you know no one, where you don't know how long you will stay, and where you will share a semiprivate room with a stranger? You pray to the good Lord. You pray that the nurses will do their job well, you pray that your incision will heal quickly, and most importantly, you pray that your roommate will be a pleasant, agreeable person.

At age seventy, I had never spent a day in a hospital except when I had my two children. Those were joyous occasions. I never asked, when am I going home? Staying at Bridgepoint would be an entirely different situation.

Two of he nurses on duty made me comfortable. They helped me put my toiletries on the nightstand and put away my tote bag in a cupboard. One nurse said they served lunch around noon. As they turned to leave, I asked them to pull back the curtain around my bed. A grey-haired Caucasian woman, sitting on the other side of the room in a wheelchair beside her bed, smiled at me.

"Hello there, I'm Patricia," she said.

"Hello, Patricia, I'm Yvonne."

"You look like a nice lady. I hope we will get along well."

Oh, boy, one of those. I'd better set this woman straight.

"I'm here for rehab. I don't know of any reason why we can't," I replied.

"I said that only because my last roommate was crazy. She was a witch. We just could not get along," Patricia said, apology heavy in her voice.

"Don't worry, Patricia, I'm the most easygoing person you'll ever meet."

We both laughed. My words smashed the ice. After that, we talked about ourselves. We had some things in common: we were the same age, we'd worked for a bank, and we were divorced. Lunch arrived. We ate and discussed how tasty the food was, compared to the food at Mt. Sinai and St. Michael's Hospital, where Patricia had her surgery. She had fallen at her home and broken several bones in her foot. She'd been at Bridgepoint for a month and knew all about the menu.

The nurses quarantined me in my room for the first seven days. I thought it rather stupid since I'd been transported directly from Mt. Sinai Hospital and had had no contact with anyone except the two patient transporters who lifted me on a sheet and swayed me from one bed to another. But as Ben Franklin once said, "An ounce of prevention is worth a pound of cure." I believe strongly in prevention.

It was at Bridgepoint that I first saw the incision on my right thigh. I almost fainted. The scar, eighteen inches long, ran from my groin, down the centre of my thigh, to about two inches below my knee. It looked like a plaited rope, with thin black stitches jutting out at intervals. The other part of my thigh, where the plastic surgeon had taken a flap, showed an incision she had stapled, not stitched like the main incision. The staples looked like a set of shark's teeth. Bridgepoint provided excellent pain management, and I thanked God for that.

* * *

The day after my seven-day quarantine ended, an Asian man walked into my room. He was thin—not an ounce of fat on his body. He had salt-and-pepper hair that bounced on his shoulders. He came over to my bed.

"Are you Yvonne?" he asked.

"Yes, I am."

"Can you confirm your date of birth, please?"

I did.

"Thank you. I just had to make sure you are the right patient. My name is Dennis, and I'm your physiotherapist."

"He's Dennis the Menace," Patricia called out from her bed. We all laughed. It seemed she had established a good rapport with Dennis.

Dennis taught me some foot exercises to do in bed. He promised to collect me to do exercises every day from Monday to Friday each week. I would have to walk to the exercise room using a walker, wearing the Zimmer brace. True to his word, Dennis returned the next day and helped me to a walker. I tried to be stoic and walked the long corridor, past several patients' rooms, past the nurses' station, to the exercise room situated at the far end on the same floor. He walked behind me with a wheelchair in case I needed to rest. Exhausted on arrival, I asked Dennis to help me sit in the wheelchair.

The exercise room was large, with one wall built entirely of windows stretching from floor to ceiling. I stared through the windows at a large part of the Toronto skyline, areas I could not see from the windows of my room. The CN Tower, the Scotia Centre, and several other skyscrapers appeared as if you could reach out and touch them. The Don Valley Parkway ran parallel to that side of the building. Lines of traffic moved on it like a funeral procession. A strip of land populated with thick shrubs separated the parkway from the river valley. The Don River, parallel to the strip of land, flowed lazily with barely a ripple. The view was spectacular.

"This view is a great incentive for me to come here and do exercises," I told Dennis.

"Yes, it's beautiful, isn't it? All our patients love it."

Dennis guided me through a series of exercises, and I did them each day. I stood and held onto a built-in rail, then kicked each foot forward, backward, and sideways, counting as I did each set. I stood on my toes, then heels, then toes and heels several times.

By the fourth week, Dennis had instructed me how to walk up and down a mini staircase with four steps, using a cane. I followed his instructions carefully—up each rung with the good foot first, down each step with the bad foot first. I liked Dennis. He was patient and careful but stern. My walking and strength improved over time.

* * *

After two weeks of calling the night nurses three or four times every night to help me to the washroom, I began to feel guilty. The day nurses had me wearing diapers with thick padding in the centres. I wondered how much urine they could absorb before it leaked onto the bed. The nurses always placed a soft green mat in the centre of the bed. I surmised that it would capture any leakage. After figuring this out, I stopped calling for the night nurse the first two times I wanted to urinate. I let it flow slowly into the diaper. My surmising proved correct; the thick padding absorbed it all, and I never felt wet or uncomfortable. For the remainder of my time in the hospital, I called the night nurse only once near the end of a shift, at about 6:00 a.m. I requested pull-ups during the days and big chunky diapers at night.

After a few weeks of observing the nurses working their twelve-hour shifts, I concluded that they truly reflected multicultural Toronto. Male and female nurses hailed from many countries and cultures, including the Philippines, India, Tibet, the Caribbean, China, and Russia. Of the entire roster that attended me and my roommates, only two nurses were Caucasians.

* * *

It had been only a month since I started Introduction to Creative Writing when I arrived at Bridgepoint. I made up quickly for the two classes I'd lost while at Mt. Sinai Hospital. Every morning after breakfast and a wash, I had the nurses help me onto a wheelchair and push me to the tall, broad windows at the front of the room. From that vantage point, I watched the traffic zipping by on Gerard Street. I watched pedestrians walking and people going in and out of the Tim Hortons coffee shop directly across the street. I observed a part of the city's skyline and the manicured lawn in front of the hospital. I also noticed that streetcars parked at the side of the street, opposite the hospital, and the drivers got out. A man dressed in what looked a like a hazmat suit entered the cars and sprayed the insides. COVID-19 precaution.

Besides watching the world go by, I dedicated hours to schoolwork. My hospital bedroom became my classroom. Every day, the nurses wheeled me over to the window and brought me my hospital table, laptop, notebook, and pencils. On the first day, we discovered that the cord on my call bell could not extend to the window where I sat. How would I call for help if I wanted to return to bed or use the washroom? Patricia listened to our conversation and promptly volunteered to use her bell to summon the nurses on my behalf if I needed help. From then onward, we were a team.

From my spot at the window, and sometimes from my bed, I booted up my laptop and read the lectures for Introduction to Creative Writing posted on York U.'s website. I took detailed notes, read all assignments, typed all the answers, and completed 99.9 percent of the exercises the professor posted. Sitting by the window, absorbing the summer sun, I found that the creative juices flowed. I became so engrossed in writing that several times, I was brought back to earth by the food delivery person standing over me with lunch or dinner.

I created haikus:

1. Pools of water stand still,
   Rippling when gently caressed by the wind
   Wetlands reflect the dazzling sun.

2. Overhead ascends a three-quarter moon,
   It appears white as newly fallen snow
   Then vanishes beneath gray clouds.

3. Wild rabbits appear early spring,
   Eating the grass and nibbling the plants
   They disappear when Winter comes.

I crafted prose poems. I concocted a short story with a first-person narrator, then rewrote it with a third-person narrator. The different perspectives were fascinating. I critiqued dozens of stories written by my peers. I created an ode to the letter *O*. I rewrote passages of books by famed authors, employing different points of view. In a show-and-tell exercise, I wrote a passage as a pure narrative, then as pure dramatization with no narration, then as a mixture of show-and-tell.

The nurses, most of them millennials, were curious about what I was doing on my laptop.

"What are you doing on that thing?" they'd ask. They probably thought I was playing games or watching movies.

"I'm doing homework for a course I'm taking at York University," I'd reply.

"No kidding! You're a student?" Big eyes, big grins.

Soon after, the nurses dubbed me "the student patient."

For each class, students had to complete four or five writing exercises. For one of the exercises, we had to select a random word and freewrite about it without stopping for ten minutes before every class. The view from my hospital room window provided fodder for this exercise. I freewrote on words including *streetcar*, *nurse*, and *pigeons*—a flock of about fifty landed on the lawn several times each day.

* * *

Staying in a hospital for two months was a lazy, boring life. The tedious, repetitious experience would have driven me insane. I thank God that He had given me the gift of writing and that I was pursuing an English degree that required a lot of writing. Whenever I wrote, I became absorbed and travelled to another galaxy. It kept me sane.

Some days, it was hard to get motivated to do my schoolwork. Some days, I felt sorry for myself because I could not walk without assistance or do anything for myself. I had to press the call button for the nurses to take me to the washroom. There were days when depression seeped in like a ghost.

One morning, I was sitting by the window, doing schoolwork as usual. My day nurse was in the room, making up my bed. A sheet of paper with some notes fell off my table and slid to the ground. I tried different ways to retrieve it, but I couldn't. Out of the blue, I burst into tears. I hadn't cried in years. The poor Pilipino nurse stopped making the bed and looked at me, stunned. She dropped the sheet, rushed over, and picked up the document.

"It's okay, Miss Yvonne. I know it's frustrating when you can't do the things you're used to, but give it time," she consoled me while rubbing my back.

I had a good cry and felt better.

I resumed my studies.

The thought of lying in bed all day like a log spurred me to get up and do my schoolwork. Besides, the room always felt cold. Sitting at the window, I enjoyed the view of nature and the warm sunshine seeping through in June and July. Whenever depression filtered in, I retrieved my little pocket Bible from the night table, read a psalm or two, and prayed. The reading and prayers always perked me up.

* * *

When Patricia learned that I am an author, our relationship strengthened. She was one of the most avid readers I'd ever met. She used a wheelchair to roam around the hospital on her own. She visited the on-site library a few times each week and borrowed two or three books at a time. Patricia read a four-hundred-page novel in two days. She also loved to be with people and spent a part of her days riding up and down the corridor, greeting other patients and catching up on gossip. She visited the lounge on our floor and watched the news on TV every day. The sad thing about her was that no one phoned or came to see her.

Patricia had to return to St. Michael's Hospital for a second surgery. The night before she departed, while her nurse prepared her for bed, I offered to pray for her. I'm no Billy Graham; I said a simple prayer, asking for the surgery and recovery to go well. Patricia was overcome with emotion that someone had prayed for her, and broke into tears. The nurse and I consoled her until she calmed down. She anticipated spending two nights at St. Michael's Hospital and hoped, with all her heart, to return to our room. Unfortunately, Bridgepoint had a different plan, and things didn't work out her way. The next evening, another woman claimed Patricia's bed after housekeeping stripped, sanitized, and remade it.

Lyn became my new roommate. She was a petite Caucasian woman with short, mousey-coloured hair and black-rimmed glasses. She had maintained a good figure at age seventy-six. We liked each other instantly. She had sarcoma cancer like me, but it was in her right arm. She had surgery to remove the tumours and kept her arm in a sling. The hospital quarantined her in the room for seven days; however, unlike me, she could walk around the room on her own. Lyn had great support from her husband, daughter, son-in-law, and grandchildren. She constantly spoke to them on her cell phone or through FaceTime on her iPad. After her quarantine ended, her husband, Howard, and her daughter visited several times. She introduced me to Howard the first time he came. After that, he brought me Iced Capps from Tim Hortons every time he came.

I did not order the hospital's expensive TV service. My roommates did not either. Megan, my daughter-in-law, gave me a little radio (bless her heart) and earbuds. Everyday, I tuned in to listen to music without disturbing my roommate. In the evenings, while we ate dinner, I removed the earbuds and turned up the volume so Lyn could also hear the news. Of course, if anything dramatic happened in Canada or the world, we discussed it.

Whenever Lyn saw me sitting near the window typing on my laptop, she asked what I was doing. She became interested in my writing after I informed her I was an author. We would invariably launch into discussions about books we'd read. Sometimes, I read pieces of my writing exercises, "Word of the Day," to her. She always gave valuable feedback.

Lyn's arm improved rapidly, and the hospital discharged her the week of July 5th. As we said our goodbyes, we promised to keep in touch. She had been an agreeable, friendly roommate indeed.

Howard came to take her home.

"Howard, do not send me any bills for the Iced Capps," I joked.

"I'll not only send you a bill, I'll add delivery charges to it," he said. He and Lyn cracked up laughing as he left the room.

After Lyn departed, I felt an emptiness. I began to yearn to go home. I knew I would miss her. The hospital did not leave me alone for long. My third roommate arrived on a stretcher later that evening. The nurses drew the curtains around her bed as the patient transporters swung her from the stretcher to bed. I couldn't see what was going on, but I heard her dishing out instructions to the nurses about what to do and what not to do. She seemed delicate and kept yelling, "Under the kneecap! Hold me under the kneecap!" every time they touched her.

At dinnertime a nurse drew back the curtains, and I saw my third roommate for the first time. She was a Caucasian woman with shoulder-length, platinum-blond hair. Her face was smooth, without wrinkles. I assessed her to be about sixty. She said hello, and told me her name was Kathy. I told her my name. The food server arrived and placed our meals on our overbed tables. Now that I had become a veteran patient, I explained the menu and meal service to her and declared that the food was good. She thanked me for the information.

By the end of the next day, I realized that Kathy was not friendly as my two previous roommates. I devoted my time to reading and writing and left it up to her to forge a friendship if and when she desired.

* * *

I had not informed the professor of my previous course that I had radiation treatment during the semester. The syllabus document for my current course, Introduction to Creative Writing, stated, "The penalty for work submitted beyond the assigned due date is a deduction of one full grade per week or part thereof." I thought the penalty was rather draconian. But the professor had every right to implement her rules. Who was I to argue against them? I sent her an email that explained that I had undergone surgery and was in a hospital. I requested her permission to submit a couple of my assignments late if need be. She gave me the green light. In the end, I did not use the exception. I submitted all of my assignments on time. The course had no final exam, but we had to do excessive writing. I wrote until my fingers became sore (I always wrote in longhand and then typed it).

The class was unique, and all students had to have a writer's notebook. In it, we had to record everything we did relating to the course. All the exercises completed, all assignments written, all critiquing of the writings of our peers, all responses to questions posed by the professor, and all responses to our classmates' replies, had to be written in the notebook chronologically. In other words, if you wanted to pass the course, you could not slack off and avoid doing the work, because, on the last day, you had to submit scanned copies of the pages of your writer's notebook or a PDF of a typed copy of everything you recorded in the notebook. Utilizing my time-management skills, I'd kept a running file of all my writings as a Word document, adding my activities each day. When the final day came to submit the notebook, I merely checked the document for grammar and spelling and then forwarded it.

The professor gave us this instruction for one of the writing exercises just before I had surgery:

> You will go for a walk to observe and then describe a landscape objectively in detailed sensory imagery. Go for a walk intentionally; your sole focus should

> be walking and experiencing the world around you. Pay close attention to the world around you with all your senses. Look up and around. Look outside yourself at the scene. Limit how much you bring yourself into the picture. You are not the subject; the setting is. This is a description exercise, showing.

Below, I described my walk:

> Walking along the paved sidewalk that runs parallel to Ashfield Drive in a suburb of Richmond Hill, a slight wind tickles the branches of the trees, most not fully in spring mode, others covered in delicate green leaves, some flowering. The air is cool and crisp. A wild rabbit hops across the sidewalk into the grass. There is no indication that the residents are up and about, the driveways are filled with cars. Only two cars motoring toward Yonge Street pass by before I turn onto a paved narrow path.
>
> It's 6:30 a.m. I enter a section of the Oak Ridges Moraine located in a residential area. This section of the moraine is bordered on one side by Ashfield Drive and the other side by North Lake Road and is separated from the road by a low metal barrier that one can easily step over. The area is wetlands populated with reeds, shrubs and a few trees. It is a habitat for birds and wild creatures. Unseen birds twittered, and bird calls filled the air. A robin with its orangey-coloured breast dives onto the path as I enter through the opened gate.
>
> A large pool of water on the left of the path ripples as a slight wind caresses it. There are ten Canada Geese at different spots, some swimming around, some standing still, others occasionally flying at each other, then landing back in the water.

The sun is brilliant as it rises in the east. To the right of the path, another pool of water stands stagnant among a sea of reeds that are dry and beige and looks like dried corn plants. They appear to be dead. The pool is murky and covered in green moss. There are no geese in it at this time.

Two grackles alight on small branches of two of three massive willow trees in the wetlands, their black feathers glistening with a blueish tinge. The trunks of the willows are gnarled and gray. The twittering and bird calls all around become louder. Several redwing blackbirds fly low into the dried reeds. Interestingly, the grass and weeds growing at the edges of the paved path are green and lush on both sides. Geese poop is strewn along the path, and one must watch where to walk. A lone goose with a white-feathered ribbon across its neck is visible now among the reeds on the right near the murky water.

Someone has dumped an empty purple Monster drink can on the grass at the edge of the path. Humans! The sun has risen higher and reflects on the water to the left, causing one to squint. In a small enclave along the path, two wooden benches facing each other are anchored into a concrete slab. It's a good spot to sit and observe the entire view of the area. Large man-made boulders separate the path from the reeds here. The orchestra of the bird song is more distinguishable—redwing blackbirds, grackles, robins, sparrows, cardinals, blue jays, and of course, the distinctive honking of the Canada geese. There is constant movement as birds dart from tree to tree and into the reeds, some landing on the path. The geese honk, and some preen themselves. Deeper into the reeds at the right, a large goose stands on a mound of dried reeds—a nest?

A birdwatcher standing among the reeds on the left, peers through a camera with a conspicuous telephoto lens set on a tripod. He wears a dark coat with a hood covering his head. He wears glasses. He takes many pictures of the geese frolicking in the water, swimming, flying, and landing. A raised boardwalk runs through the moraine from the North Lake Road end to Ashfield Drive. It has two paths. Standing on one of the boardwalk paths, I spot a small creature, maybe a chipmunk or a badger, swimming in the water. It goes through a small tunnel built into a concrete divider that separates the pool of water on the left into two.

The birdwatcher collects his camera and tripod and walks by me on the boardwalk. He does not speak. He is an Asian man. He goes to the right side and spends a few minutes taking more pictures. He passes me again. This time he says, "Did you see the baby ducks?" I say "No. Where are they?" He continues walking, and I'm thinking, he is calling baby geese baby ducks!

Chlorophyll is returning to the reeds on the left. Green shoots dispersed among the dried stalks are visible here. Dozens of redwing blackbirds fly from reed to reed, landing and balancing on the spindly stalks.

By 7:30 a.m., the sun no longer reflects directly on the water in the moraine. A white-haired woman dressed in a puffer coat walks by with a magnificent black and white dog on a leash. "He's a border collie," she says when asked about his pedigree. Heading toward the exit on Ashfield Drive, I see three mallard ducks—their bright green heads distinctive—swimming in the water on the left. The Asian man was probably correct; there could have been baby mallard ducks in the water.

I leave the moraine to a chorus of birdsong—geese honking, birds twittering, and birds calling. A little black squirrel dashes onto the path and scampers up a tree on the sidewalk. A few flowering plants on the circumference of the moraine bloom white flowers that look like long-grain rice clustered among their tiny red leaves. Three large willow trees now have yellow-green leaves. Walking along the paved sidewalk back to my home, I observe the side yard of the house at the corner is covered every inch with dandelions, their yellow flowers slightly opened in the early morning.

The professor wrote this comment when she marked my paper: "Absolutely stunning work."

* * *

I visited my surgeon for my third checkup on July 20th. He examined my incision and assured me that it was healing well, and faster than he had expected, considering that the thigh had received radiation. The incision had two small "hot spots"—one three inches, the other six inches above the knee—that had not yet healed. They were shallow, and the surgeon had no concerns about them.

I'd developed a special relationship with the nurses. I said goodbye to my favourites on my return from my surgeon, knowing my discharge was imminent. I presented them with little blue thank-you cards penned with personal notes. I experienced what Juliet must have felt when she said, "Parting is such sweet sorrow."

Bridgepoint Health discharged me the next day. I had spent two months there and was excited to be going home. For the final time, the nurses completed their usual checks—vitals—and administered medications. They assured me that the two hot spots in my incision were healing nicely, so I did not require a visiting nurse to dress them. They gave me packages of gauze, bandages, and a bottle of saline solution, and instructed me to wash my hands every day and use fresh gauze to clean the wounds with the saline, then cover them with bandages.

CHAPTER TWENTY-TWO

No Place Like Home

"It's a funny thing coming home. Nothing changes. Everything looks the same, feels the same, even smells the same. You realized what's changed is you."

—F. SCOTT FITZGERALD

Rob came to my hospital room and gathered up my few personal effects, including my laptop. He also collected a walker and a cane I had purchased from one of the stores recommended by Bridgepoint. The cane was a flashy pink number, lightweight but sturdy. He helped me into a wheelchair and pushed it to the elevator, then down to the underground garage. Rob is six foot four and sturdy. I felt like an infant being taken care of by a parent. How the tides had turned! Andrea, one of my favourite nurses, who had painlessly removed forty stitches from my thigh in one session, accompanied us to the car so she could return the wheelchair to the floor. Rob helped me into his car as if I were precious cargo.

At 11:00 a.m., Rob backed his car onto the driveway of my home in Richmond Hill to allow me room to maneuver.

"Wait here, Mom, don't do anything yet," he said and rushed to unlock the front door, then removed my walker from the back seat. He brought the walker to the passenger side and waited for me to get out of the car. The Toyota Corolla was low, and it took me several attempts to get out. I began to learn how difficult things would become without the full use of my right leg. Rob waited patiently until I felt comfortable enough to stand on the driveway. I walked, using the walker, to the front step and stopped. What did Dennis, the therapist, teach me about ascending stairs and steps? "You put your good foot first, then the bad foot." With his voice echoing in my head, I followed those instructions and mounted the single step, then rose up onto the front porch. Rob stayed beside me all the way like a mama bear protecting its cub. He threw open the front door, and I entered my home for the first time after spending two months in the hospital.

The hardwood floor gleamed in the hallway.

"Peace be onto the house," I said. "My goodness! I could comb my hair using the floor as a mirror."

"Megan and I cleaned it for you on Sunday," Rob said.

"Thanks to both of you. I do appreciate it."

As I walked by the stairs, I stopped to look up at the steps. Six steps, deep and wide, led to a landing where I had placed a deacon's bench, a suggestion by my real estate agent when I had bought the house. "Put a bench on the first landing in case you get tired when you reach there," she'd said. I had searched diligently and found the perfect bench, with storage space beneath the seat, in a small furniture store. The salesman said it was the last of its kind because the carpenter who made it had died from cancer. I am pleased to report that during the eleven years I lived in the house, I had never sat on the bench after climbing those six steps. There were three steps after the first landing, another landing, then six more steps to reach the second floor. The right side of the stairs had a sturdy oak railing, but there was no railing on the left. I passed the stairs, walked into the living room, and sat on the sofa.

"Do you plan to go upstairs to your bedroom?" Rob asked.

"No, I'm too scared of falling. Although Dennis taught me how to go up and down stairs, it's one thing to practice on a mini staircase and another to do it on an actual staircase."

The surgeon had removed the muscles in my right thigh where the tumours were embedded and inserted a metal rod to strengthen it, but my leg remained weak. Walking with a walker was the safest way to move around. I didn't want to risk falling and decided not to go upstairs to my bedroom.

"I'm staying downstairs for the first few weeks to get some strength back in my right leg," I said.

"You can't sleep on the sofa for that long, Mom. I'll get a single bed and set it up in the living room for you."

"That's very thoughtful of you, son. Thank you."

"No problem, I have only one mother." He hugged me tightly, then dashed off to collect medications the doctor at the hospital had prescribed. The doctor had forwarded the prescription to a pharmacy near my house.

Minutes after Rob left, Megan, his wife, arrived. I thanked her for the cleaning job. She offered to purchase any groceries needed and suggested I make a list. I lumbered over to the fridge to check the shelves. They were bare as Old Mother Hubbard's cupboard. I knew I would not be able to cook any meals for some time, and included enough Lean Cuisine meals in the list to last a week. Rob returned with the medications, then left for a half day of work. Megan headed for the supermarket located just across the property fence at the front of the townhouse complex.

The doorbell rang at noon. I hobbled along with my walker to see who had arrived. I opened the door, and there stood Emilio, the husband of Maria, a member of my Italian posse.

"Hi there! Welcome home. I've brought food for you, my dear," he said.

He carried two boxes without covers in his arms. Emilio came inside and unpacked the boxes, placing the contents on the kitchen counter. They were packaged individual meals, labelled and ready for me to eat. I read some of the labels—veal, chicken, Italian sausage, and salmon. Looking through the plastic containers, I observed that each meal contained meat, vegetables, and a starch. There was also a large container with a field salad.

"Oh, Emilio, your wife is too kind. I spoke to her yesterday and told her I was coming home, but she never said a word about the food. Please thank her for me. I so appreciate it," I said as my eyes welled up with tears.

"The food is from Maria and Michelina. I'm just the delivery man," Emilio said.

He helped me to stack the meals in the freezer. There were enough to last two weeks.

"Maria said to call her whenever you run low, and she'll send some more," he said.

"Thank you for the delivery, Emilio. I'll call her later."

After Emilio departed, I wanted to get down on my knees, but my eighteen-inch incision and stiff knees would not allow it. I sat on the sofa and looked around the house. I was in my own home, in my own space, alone, but not truly alone. There would be no nurses trooping in and out, no physiotherapist coming to take me to the exercise room, no bantering back and forth with a roommate, and no food service people arriving with breakfast, lunch, and dinner. I felt happy as a pig in the mud. The freezer was stocked with the food Emilio brought, and soon Megan would return with the groceries. I knew that fellowship would build as family and friends began to telephone and pop in for visits. I called Maria the next day. Michelina visited me twice and brought similar amounts of food each time.

Sitting on the sofa, I closed my eyes and prayed to my Creator. I thanked Him for health—yes, health, for, despite the surgery and all the pain that went with it, I felt well in my mind and body. I thanked Him for always looking out for me, and for providing kind, loving friends like Maria and Michelina, and for family. I felt truly blessed.

Megan returned with the groceries. She had to stack the boxes of Lean Cuisine meals in the door compartment of the freezer. The nutritious Italian meals had taken up all the regular space. I knew the Lean Cuisine dinners would remain in the freezer uneaten for some time. Megan dashed upstairs and brought down pillows, sheets, and towels from my bedroom. She made the sofa comfortable for me to sleep on, then headed home after she felt satisfied that I had settled and would be okay alone for the night.

Two days later, Rob removed the coffee table from the living room and placed it in the basement. He assembled a single bed in its place. I lived downstairs for the next few months, going upstairs to shower occasionally, but only with the help of the personal support worker (PSW) who came twice each week to assist with my personal care.

* * *

Three weeks remained to complete Introduction to Creative Writing and thus complete the degree. I created a workstation in the living room, using the largest of four cherrywood nesting tables for my desk and an armchair from the dining table for my seat. I placed my laptop on the nesting table along with my writing paraphernalia. The location was perfect for my "office" because an electrical outlet was nearby for recharging the laptop and cell phone.

I spent many hours sitting at the nesting table each day, reading the final lectures, completing the writing exercises, responding to the questions posed by the professor, and replying to the responses my classmates posted. On the morning of August 8th, the final day of the course, I submitted my writer's notebook document, consisting of thirty-five pages, to my professor. All students had to create a portfolio of their work and send it to the professor the next day. In her instructions, she demanded, "A polished presentation of your best literary writing consisting of 15-20 pages double spaced." She also required a two-page self-evaluation from us. I chose some of what I considered my best writings for my portfolio—haikus, sonnets, prose poems, freewriting exercises, and short stories. I included my walk description because the professor liked it. I wrote a two-page self-evaluation stating honestly how I felt about the course and that I'd learned a lot. After editing for grammatical and spelling errors, I submitted my portfolio and self-evaluation on the evening of August 8th, a day early—my last hurrah.

This time, I waited anxiously to receive my mark. Would it be a B that would lower my GPA? Would it be an A that would maintain my GPA and propel me into summa cum laude graduating status?

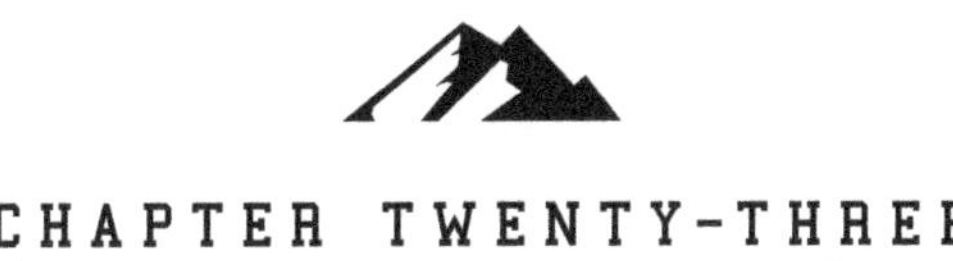

CHAPTER TWENTY-THREE

The Graduate

"The roots of education are bitter, but the fruit is sweet."
—ARISTOTLE

In my world of setting goals, making plans, and working on those plans, there is nothing quite as exhilarating and satisfying as achieving those goals. Back in the 1980s, when I'd set a goal to travel to six of the seven continents, some friends thought the idea rather far-fetched. I not only touched down on six continents, but I also visited some of them several times as I explored a different country on each journey. Those achievements were exciting, and I took pleasure in ticking off the countries I'd visited from my bucket list.

Earning an English degree became another of my goals and the reason for this story. I wrote and submitted my last paper for the final course to complete the degree in August 2021. I waited a few weeks, then reviewed my student record online. My marks had been tabulated and audited, and York University confirmed that I had earned a bachelor's degree in English.

I thought about York U.'s motto, *Tentanda via* (the way must be tried), and gushed with pride as I recalled how hard I had *tried the way*. Langston Hughes, the famed African American writer and poet, wrote the poem "Mother to Son," which metaphorically articulated my struggle as I tried the way:

> Well, son, I'll tell you:
> Life for me ain't been no crystal stair.
> It's had tacks in it,
> And splinters,
> And boards torn up,
> And places with no carpet on the floor—
> Bare…

I had climbed hard stairs too. It had tacks in it. In fact, I would say it had long, sharp nails in it, but I never turned back and never gave up.

When York U. stopped the YRT (my means of commute) from coming on the campus grounds as it had done for many years, I found a way to walk from the bus stop through sunshine, sleet, and snow and stayed the course. When the workers of York U. went on strike twice, causing the addition of a year to the time I'd scheduled to earn my degree, I stayed the course. When York U. locked down the campus because of COVID-19 and switched all classes to online, which was not my preference, I completed the remainder of my classes in that format and stayed the course. When I could not register for a necessary summer course to fulfill the requirement of an English major, I found a way and stayed the course. When I was diagnosed with sarcoma cancer and slated for five weeks of radiation treatment for five days each week, I arranged a new, convenient accommodation and stayed the course. When I had surgery on my right thigh and remained in the hospital for two months, I continued my studies from my hospital bed and stayed the course. When I returned home from the hospital and could only walk with a walker, I continued my studies and wrote my final paper three weeks later by staying the course. I overcame every barrier, every obstacle, every hurdle, and found a way to continue to climb the mountain until I reached the summit.

* * *

In early September, as I was waiting for the results of my final course, anxious to learn if I would graduate summa cum laude, something terrible happened to a small hole in the incision in my thigh. I had followed all the instructions that the nurses gave me at Bridgepoint Health about caring for two hot spots in the incision. My surgeon had instructed me to leave the areas uncovered during the daytime, allowing them to air. I had adhered to his instructions. After two weeks at home, the hot spot six inches above my knee developed a scab and closed. The area healed but remained tender to the touch. The other hot spot, three inches above the knee, remained raw and open. I was shocked when it began to ooze pus with an odour. I called my surgeon, but he was away on vacation. I took a taxi to a drop-in clinic near my home. I was the second-to-last patient for the day, and when the doctor finally inspected my wound, she scared the daylights out of me.

"You have an infection deep down in the wound, and with the nail" (that was what she called the metal post) "in your thigh, the infection could travel down to your bone. You need to go to the Emerge at the hospital right away." With that, she left me in the small examination room.

A fog enveloped my brain; I couldn't think straight. I had been through so much in the past five months, beginning with the radiation treatment. Was I going to lose my leg? How would I get to Emerge from the clinic? I telephoned the taxi company I'd used to get to the clinic, the only number I had at that time. A dispatcher said a taxi would arrive in fifteen minutes. In the meantime, the clinic closed for the day. I sauntered with my walker down the hallway and exited the building.

Fifteen minutes turned into thirty minutes, and the taxi did not arrive. I called the taxi company for the third time to say the car had not arrived. I had been standing outside the clinic leaning against a wall, holding onto a walker. The dispatcher hung up on me. With the clinic closed, I had no further access to it. What could I do? Suddenly, I remembered Peggy, a friend who lived in the neighbourhood. I phoned her, and within ten minutes, she arrived. Peggy had telephoned several times to check on me since I returned home after the surgery, but because of COVID-19, she had not visited me. Her eyes opened wide when she saw me leaning over my walker. She helped me into her car and placed the walker in the trunk. I was seething with rage at the taxi dispatcher all the way to my area hospital.

"Can you believe the nerve of that guy? He hung up on me, a customer!"

"Never mind, my dear, don't waste your energy on anger. Focus on your health," Peggy consoled me.

She deposited me at the entrance of the emergency department at 5:45 p.m.

"If they don't admit you, call me when you're ready to go home, and I'll come back for you," she said.

"Thank you so much, Peggy, but if it's late, I won't call."

Entering the emergency department in the hospital makes you feel that there is no such thing as an emergency. The procedure was lengthy and drawn out as I moved from registration to triage to registration again. I phoned Rob to tell him about my situation. I heard him gasp through the phone, but he remained calm. He asked me to keep him updated. Several hours later, a doctor came to see me. He ordered a CT scan of my thigh. A porter pushed me in a wheelchair to the imaging department.

Waiting for the CT scan results felt like I was living in a nightmare. All kinds of thoughts raced through my mind. What would they find? Had the infection touched my bone as the clinic doctor had insinuated? At 10:30 p.m., the emergency doctor I'd seen earlier returned to see me. The doctor at the clinic had scared me enough, but he added kindling to the fire. The CT scan showed a lot of fluid had pooled in my thigh. The doctors could not determine if it was blood or something else. He wanted to refer me to one of their orthopedic surgeons. After absorbing the information, I spoke softly but decisively to him.

"Doctor, please know that I have nothing against this hospital, but if anything has to be done to my leg, I don't want it to be done here. My surgeon and my records are at Mt. Sinai. I would like to be sent there. I know my surgeon is on vacation, but there is always a backup doctor."

The doctor looked at me, and an expression of understanding covered his face.

"All right, wait here, and I will call Mt. Sinai."

He left me in the cubicle and returned ten minutes later to say that the backup doctor asked that I report to their Emerge the next day by 9:00 a.m. He gave me a note with the name of the doctor at Mt. Sinai and the details of the CT scan. He did not admit me to the hospital but sent me home. It was almost midnight and too late to call Peggy. The hospital had a designated number for taxis on call. I called for one, and within five minutes, the car arrived. On the way home, I sent Rob a text, asking him to take me to Mt. Sinai's Emerge the next day.

Rob deposited me at the emergency entrance of Mt. Sinai and departed. The emergency procedure, similar to that of my area hospital, was overly long and wearisome. At 3:30 p.m., a porter wheeled me in a wheelchair to an overflow room on the seventeenth floor. The consulting doctor arrived with a female doctor thirty minutes later. She inspected the wound, measured its depth, and cleaned it with a brown antiseptic. She packed it with six inches of gauze soaked in the same antiseptic, then placed a waterproof bandage on it. I could not believe that the small hole in the incision was deep enough to hold so much gauze. I had no fever or chills and did not feel ill, so the consulting doctor did not admit me to the hospital. He instructed me to see my surgeon when he returned in three days and sent me home.

I called my surgeon early the day he returned to work to make an appointment.

"It's the middle of the Jewish holidays, and the doctor is not seeing many patients. The earliest appointment I can give you is the sixteenth," the assistant said.

"That date will not do. I have to see him today or tomorrow the latest. Listen to me, I have packing in my wound and a bandage that must be changed. It cannot wait a whole week," I said adamantly.

"Okay, Mrs. Blackwood, I will make arrangements for a nurse to visit you at home, and I'll book the sixteenth for your appointment with the doctor."

"Thank you. I'm glad you understand my position."

A nurse arrived at my home the next day. She removed the packing from the wound, cleaned it, and applied fresh gauze and a bandage. She returned a few more times before my appointment with the surgeon.

Thirteen days after the emergency doctor at my area hospital scared me with the information that there was a lot of liquid pooling in my thigh, I saw my surgeon. He examined the wound, squeezed it, and said it had no pus. He assured me that it was healing fine.

"What about all that fluid the CT scan showed pooling in my thigh?" I asked, knowing he would have received the report from my area hospital. Besides, doctors have access to medical information through the hospital system.

"I don't think you should worry about it. Remember that when we took out the muscles with the tumors, it left a big hole in your thigh. The hole is like a vacuum; it attracts liquid in the body," my surgeon explained.

I accepted his explanation. After all, he would have seen many similar cases. The nurse cleaned the wound and redressed it. I went home feeling confident that it would soon heal, and I could now focus on the rest of my recovery. Nurses came to my home every day to dress the wound, but it would not heal. I began to feel intermittent, pulsating pains in my knee that I had never felt before, and the leg became heavier and stiffer. I contacted my surgeon and met with him for an appointment. I told him emphatically that something was wrong with my leg. He grudgingly agreed to order an MRI, stating that he knew they would not find anything, but "I'll do it for your peace of mind."

* * *

In October, I received an invitation via email from the Convocation Office to attend "Grad Days" by making an appointment. York U. had decided that while COVID-19 still raged and the campus remained under lockdown, they would host in-person Grad Days under a rigid COVID-19 protocol. There would be no in-person convocation ceremony; however, they would hold an online ceremony on November 2nd. Attendees of Grad Days would collect their diplomas, be gowned, and have a mortarboard placed on their heads, and the university's photographers would take their graduation pictures.

How could I turn down such a wonderful invitation? Grad Days would be the culmination of the years I had worked and the effort I'd expended to earn my English degree. How could I allow sarcoma cancer surgery and the incision in my right thigh that refused to heal to deter me from personally collecting my prize? York U. would not deliver diplomas to anyone except students in person. If I did not attend Grad Days, they would mail it to my address on file. Collecting my diploma from the mailbox would be disappointing, dissatisfying, and so disheartening. I had looked forward to walking across the stage at Convocation Hall and collecting my diploma while friends and family cheered me on. Since this was the best the university could provide under COVID-19 conditions, I would take it.

When I began to study for the English degree, I was healthy and vibrant, doing everything on my own. I used to walk more than a mile to get to some classes. My circumstances significantly changed since surgery in May 2021. Now I could not walk outside unaccompanied—my right leg could buckle, and I would fall. I had a long incision in my right thigh with a small area that would not heal. I used a walker to go everywhere—to the kitchen, to the bathroom, to open my front door. But I was adamant that the handicap would not stop me from attending Grad Days and personally collecting my diploma, my prize. I made an appointment with the Convocation Office for a Saturday afternoon. They allowed me two guests. I chose my son Rob, my chauffeur, and Maria, a member of my Chinese posse. Maria felt extremely honoured that she was the chosen guest and was excited to help me throughout the process.

The New Student Centre was the venue for Grad Days. I had visited the centre a few times while on campus by walking along a path from another building; however, I could not direct Rob to the building. He drove around for a while, trying to find it. He eventually found the building by approaching it from the rear. A steep ramp constructed with rough, bumpy concrete led to the back doors. I ascended it with my walker with much difficulty, only to find the doors locked. The Grad Days organizers had bolted all the doors to the centre except the main front door because of COVID-19 protocol. Maria and Rob walked beside me as we descended the ramp and travelled along a lengthy side path. I arrived at the front door exhausted.

The people guarding the front door of the New Student Centre asked us 101 COVID-19 questions and checked our vaccine status before they allowed us inside. Of course, they had included the details about the procedure with my invitation, so we were prepared.

I walked gingerly with my walker along a path covered with a red carpet that wound its way from one station to another. At the first station, a man sprang from behind the counter and helped me put on the black gown and red hood. He placed the black mortarboard on my head, with the tassel falling the right way. I had purchased my graduation garb instead of renting it—a memorabilia for my grandsons.

I continued along the red carpet to the second station, where a student handed me my diploma in a white envelope. There was nothing dramatic about the delivery, thanks to COVID-19. I checked the document to make sure it had the correct spelling of my name. The words "Magna Cum Laude" were printed in red above the chancellor's signature and the date. I was graduating with "great honour." I broke into a wide grin that a Cheshire cat would have had difficulty competing with. Maria whipped out her cell phone and took some photos at that moment. I commanded her not to include my walker in the pictures. When I reviewed the photographs later, there it was! The silver appliance with two front wheels and two red buttons on the crossbar, used to collapse it for storage, stood beside me.

I moved on to the third station. Four photographers stood waiting. The first one offered to take my pictures and asked me to stand before a large red frame. I explained that I could stand only for a short time without my walker and handed it to Rob. The photographer quickly took two pictures, one with me holding up the diploma and one standing with my hands at my side, smiling broadly. He then asked Rob and Maria to pose with me and took two more photos. A student at a nearby table called me over. She gave me a red shopping bag embossed with York U.'s logo. It contained two 2021 graduation pins, a red graduation cardboard box, a hand-flick confetti stick, a chocolate bar, and some brochures.

I prepared to leave the New Student Centre and told one of the organizers that the path via the front door was too long and difficult for me to walk. Could we exit through the back door? She stared at my walker, and after consulting with another person, led me to the back door. Rob, Maria, and I walked down the same ramp we had climbed earlier. It was a much shorter route. Halfway down, Rob and Maria stopped to take some outdoor pictures of me in my cap and gown. They had taken only a couple when a few raindrops splattered on my arm.

Rob dashed to get his car from a nearby parking lot and brought it close to the ramp. A minute after I entered the car, the rain began to pour, pelting the roof and windows. I watched sheets of white water slanting against the windshield, and a peaceful mood rained on me. I had put on my graduation cap and gown, collected my diploma, and taken official photographs. With that, my Grad Day was over. The rain was a shower of blessing. The sun came out again soon after.

I had not spoken to my father about the progression of my studies from the day I told him about my plans to attend university, and he'd indicated disapproval and lack of interest. The moment I arrived home, I telephoned him. Now ninety-six, he remained as sharp as a scalpel.

"Dad, I did it! I got the degree. I've just returned from the campus, and I have the diploma with me."

I wanted to brag about my achievement, to show him that his negative attitude toward my attending university in my old age had not deterred me one iota.

"Well, child," he said, "you have the Jackson blood in you. You wanted to do it, and you did. God bless you."

"Thanks, Dad," I said.

What else could I say? If he only knew the ordeal I had been through to earn the degree. But I would not burden him with such details. I did not burden anyone with the details. I share them now to encourage my fellow seniors with the words of Pearl Bailey, "Go for it,"

CHAPTER TWENTY-FOUR

Degree Conferred

"Success is no accident. It is hard work, perseverance, learning, studying, sacrifice and most of all, love of what you are doing or learning to do."

—PELÉ

My surgeon telephoned me two weeks after I had done the MRI he had grudgingly agreed to and said that he planned to reopen the incision in my thigh and clean up inside the wound; *debride* was the term he used. I should report to Mt. Sinai's emergency department when he called again. He never explained what the MRI had shown that prompted his response. I did not care. As long as he did something about my leg, that was all that mattered.

* * *

I reported to Mt. Sinai's emergency department on the last day of October. The surgeon performed a second surgery on my leg on November 1st. On the day I attended Grad Days on York U.'s campus, the day I was gowned, capped, and photographed and collected my diploma, a student reminded me that there would be no in-person convocation ceremony; however, an online ceremony would be on YouTube on November 2nd. On that day, while lying in a hospital bed, hooked up to a drip delivering powerful antibiotics, I watched my convocation ceremony on my cell phone.

Life can take such unusual twists and turns. I had only used my cell phone for urgent calls while away from home, preferring to use my landline for all regular calls. It accounted for why my classmates never saw me using a cell phone on campus. Whatever I had to talk about could wait until I returned home. But my stay in a hospital for two months changed my cell phone usage. I had gotten used to communicating by cell phone, so watching the ceremony on it was not a stretch.

The ceremony incorporated all the usual pomp and pageantry: A bagpiper, dressed in full Scottish regalia, played his pipe. A beadle marched with the mace and placed it on a small stand. The president and other faculty members, dressed in ceremonial robes, delivered speeches. The chancellor, Greg Sorbara, dressed in an official black and cream robe, delivered this message:

> *Congratulations, class of 2021!*
>
> *Earning a university degree is an extraordinary achievement at any time, but it is all the more remarkable during a global pandemic.*
>
> *The determination and resolve that you have shown throughout your time at York University, and over the past year and a half, in particular, are confirmation that you have the confidence and drive to take on whatever challenges might await you in the future.*
>
> *As a proud alumnus myself, I know how valuable a degree from York can be. York is widely recognized as a progressive university with innovative programming, world-class teaching*

and instruction, and an unwavering commitment to social justice. My learning experience at York equipped me with the knowledge and skills I needed to build a career focused on serving the public and striving for the greater good. I hope that your experience will be equally as fulfilling and transformative.

I know today is different from what you may have imagined, and that the world you are entering is full of uncertainties. History has shown us that times of great uncertainty are often times of rare opportunity—the opportunity for positive change in our lives and the world around us. I encourage you to draw on the strong foundations you have built at York to help create a brighter future for all of us.

It is my great pleasure to welcome you to the York alumni community and to wish you all the best in your future endeavours.

The chancellor was spot on when he said, "I know today is different from what you may have imagined." If he only knew about my story! Knowing there would not be an in-person convocation, I had made plans to watch the ceremony from home with my girlfriend, Gloria. We intended to banter back and forth about the event and drink a toast with a glass of champagne when they called my name. Things did not work out that way. There I was in a hospital bed, alone, watching the ceremony on a small screen.

After the chancellor ended his speech, the dean invited him to officially confer the degrees on the graduates.

He said these words:

As chancellor of York University, and by the authority of the power vested in me, I hereby confer upon you the degrees to which you have demonstrated your entitlement to the satisfaction of the Senate, with

> *such title, honour, duties, rights and privileges as are proper to them.*

After that, a woman with a clear, distinctive voice called the names of every graduating student from every faculty. She stated the wording of their degrees, including any distinctions. The information flashed on the screen with pictures of the students if they had submitted one.

I was ecstatic when I heard my name and saw my picture. The words on the screen read:

> Yvonne Eugennie Blackwood
> Bachelor of Arts
> English
> *Magna Cum Laude*
> Faculty of Liberal Arts & Professional Studies
> YorkU

Tentanda via. Amen. I had tried the way, climbed the mountain, stayed the course, kept the faith, reached the summit, and collected the prize. My studies at York U. were over. Now my health would be the focus.

Reader's Guide Questions

1. Did you enjoy the book? Why or why not?
2. How did Blackwood feel when she explored the university campus just before she began her studies and saw the young students hanging out in the corridors?
3. The writer usually drove everywhere. Do you think it was a tough decision to take the bus to school every time she had classes? What were the advantages? What are your impressions about public transportation?
4. It must have been difficult for the writer to scale back on her social life to attend university. What are some of the things she gave up?
5. It seems that the first time the writer felt out of touch was attending her first class and a student beside her used his cell phone to take a picture of the professor's slide on the overhead. What went through her mind then?
6. Blackwood had a reality check when she received a C+ for her first essay. How did she process it? Later, she received first prize for her first sonnet, albeit only three students took on the challenge. How did she feel? Did this win help to motivate her to aim for As?
7. The course Understanding Food is filled with valuable information. Would you recommend it to seniors and others?

8. The author mentioned that summer courses are hard, but to complete the degree within the timeframe set, she had to do one every year. What are some things you learned about summer courses?
9. Blackwood's great love for flora and fauna exuded from her descriptions. How much do you enjoy them during your summers or in retirement?
10. The chapter on Literature and Drugs was fascinating, but it seems Blackwood did not plan to take that course. What are some key benefits of doing that course?
11. Was there specific messages or themes in the book? Did any chapter or passage stand out that gave you an "a-ha!" moment about the topic?
12. In the chapter Peers, Blackwood mentioned that besides academic learning, she wanted to learn about them all along. What would you wish to learn about millennial students?
13. The chapter on Environmental Pollution was detailed and most informative, not just for senior citizens, but for everyone. What did you think about the author's research? Were the sources credible? Why do you think it was important for Blackwood to include the topic in the memoir?
14. Many of us have never been hospitalized, and if so, not for as long as the writer. What are some positive things she learned about a lengthy hospital stay?
15. Blackwood stated that her world stood still when she received the cancer diagnosis, yet we gather that she stayed positive throughout her illness. What are your thoughts on how she managed this?
16. There was no in-person convocation ceremony to attend because of the COVID-19 pandemic. "Grad Days" allowed students to go on campus to be gowned, capped, collect their diplomas, and have their photographs taken. Blackwood was ill and using a walker to move around. Why was it so important to her to go on campus and collect her diploma?

17. Would you recommend this book to other readers? Would you recommend it to your close friends and family members? Why or why not?
18. If you could talk to the author, what burning question would you want to ask?

Acknowledgements

Throughout my writing life, dating back to publishing my first book in 2000—fact, from my lowly birth—I've been fortunate and blessed to have the support of many people. During the challenging time of going back to school, illness, and writing this memoir, strong support swept in from several directions. If I've overlooked some names do forgive me.

A big thank you to family members who visited, called, and kept me in their prayers: Robert Blackwood, Michele Blackwood, Carol Blackwood, Donna and Pauline Benjamin, Hermine Suhr, Yvonne Komlenovich, Megan Scott, Triscott and Mary-Lou Scott.

I am extremely grateful to members of my wonderful church family who phoned, prayed, and or visited with gifts to boot: Pastor Paul Sadler, Grace Marcoccia, Sam and Nana Appiah, Guy and Anne-Marie St. Louis, Caroline Clement, Stephanie Clement, Jennifer Clement-Schlimm, Dirk Schlimm, Lynn Keats, Monica and Ken Durant, Pulie Essau, Keith and Mary Newallo.

Some of my high school friends have remained close over the years, and they called regularly or visited: Etaine Smith, Deloris & Fitzroy Wood, Carl Randall, Patricia Curnow, Paul Gunter. I thank you.

My amazing Italian posse called regularly and sent lots of food: Maria Racco, Emilio Racco, Michelina DiCarlo. I thank you.

My Chinese posse called regularly and visited: Maria Wong, Ean Lim. Thank you

My new BFFs Edith and Michael Lorimer, you provided accommodation, nurtured me, and allowed me space to continue by studies during my entire radiation treatment. I am eternally grateful to you both.

My exceptional colleagues from the banking industry called, prayed, and some visited bearing gifts: Jean Brandon, Lavern Sinkia, Shanty Pyrau, Juliet D'andrade, Claudia Small, Jennifer Thornhill, Lyn White, Pauline McKitty-Robinson. I am so grateful to you.

My friends from the community who called regularly: Peggy Francis, Adlin McFarlane, Cherita Girvan-Campbell, Pat O'Connor, Connie Foster, Gloria Wilson-Forbes, Errol Townshend, Nina Mawji. Thank you.

Thank you to my Beta readers: Gloria Wilson-Forbes and Connie Foster. Gloria wrote, "In general this book is about resilience and creativity. These character traits can be applied at any age. This is a book for all ages not just Seniors."

"A big thank you to my editor Marcia Trahan for catching the errors and for enlightening me on The Chicago Manual Style."